Imaging of Movement Disorders

Guest Editors

TAREK A. YOUSRY, Dr med Habil
ANDREW J. LEES, MD

NEUROIMAGING CLINICS OF NORTH AMERICA

www.neuroimaging.theclinics.com

Consulting Editor
SURESH K. MUKHERJI, MD

February 2010 • Volume 20 • Number 1

SAUNDERS an imprint of ELSEVIER, Inc.

W.B. SAUNDERS COMPANY
A Division of Elsevier Inc.

1600 John F. Kennedy Boulevard ● Suite 1800 ● Philadelphia, Pennsylvania 19103-2899

http://www.theclinics.com

NEUROIMAGING CLINICS OF NORTH AMERICA Volume 20, Number 1
February 2010 ISSN 1052-5149, ISBN 13: 978-1-4377-1242-1

Editor: Joanne Husovski
Developmental Editor: Donald Mumford

Neuroimaging Clinics of North America (ISSN 1052-5149) is published quarterly by Elsevier Inc., 360 Park Avenue South, New York, NY 10010-1710. Months of issue are February, May, August, and November. Business and editorial offices: 1600 John F. Kennedy Blvd., Suite 1800, Philadelphia, PA 19103-2899. Business and editorial offices: 6277 Sea Harbor Drive, Orlando, FL 32887-4800. Periodicals postage paid at New York, NY, and additional mailing offices. Subscription prices are USD 293 per year for US individuals, USD 415 per year for US institutions, USD 150 per year for US students and residents, USD 339 per year for Canadian individuals, USD 520 per year for Canadian institutions, USD 431 per year for international individuals, USD 520 per year for international institutions and USD 215 per year for Canadian and foreign students and residents. To receive student/resident rate, orders must be accompanied by name of affiliated institution, date of term, and the *signature* of program/residency coordinator on institution letterhead. Orders will be billed at individual rate until proof of status is received. Foreign air speed delivery is included in all *Clinics* subscription prices. All prices are subject to change without notice. POSTMASTER: Send address changes to *Neuroimaging Clinics of North America*, Elsevier Health Sciences Division, Subscription Customer Service, 3251 Riverport Lane, Maryland Heights, MO 63043. Telephone: 1-800-654-2452 (U.S. and Canada); 314-447-8871 (outside U.S. and Canada). Fax: 314-447-8029. E-mail: journalscustomerservice-usa@elsevier.com (for print support); journalsonlinesupport-usa@elsevier.com (for online support).

Reprints. For copies of 100 or more of articles in this publication, please contact the Commercial Reprints Department, Elsevier Inc., 360 Park Avenue South, New York, NY 10010-1710. Tel.: 212-633-3812; Fax: 212-462-1935; E-mail: reprints@elsevier.com.

Neuroimaging Clinics of North America is covered by *Excerpta Medical/EMBASE,* the RSNA Index of Imaging Literature, *MEDLINE/PubMed (Index Medicus),* MEDLINE/MEDLARS, SciSearch, Research Alert, and Neuroscience Citation Index.

Cover image © Lydia Gregg 2009.

Printed and bound by CPI Group (UK) Ltd, Croydon, CR0 4YY

Transferred to Digital Print 2011

GOAL STATEMENT

The goal of *Neuroimaging Clinics of North America* is to keep practicing radiologists and radiology residents up to date with current clinical practice in radiology by providing timely articles reviewing the state of the art in patient care.

ACCREDITATION

The *Neuroimaging Clinics of North America* is planned and implemented in accordance with the Essential Areas and Policies of the Accreditation Council for Continuing Medical Education (ACCME) through the joint sponsorship of the University of Virginia School of Medicine and Elsevier. The University of Virginia School of Medicine is accredited by the ACCME to provide continuing medical education for physicians.

The University of Virginia School of Medicine designates this educational activity for a maximum of 15 *AMA PRA Category 1 Credits*™ for each issue, 60 credits per year. Physicians should only claim credit commensurate with the extent of their participation in the activity.

The American Medical Association has determined that physicians not licensed in the US who participate in this CME activity are eligible for a maximum of 15 *AMA PRA Category 1 Credits*™ for each issue, 60 credits per year.

Credit can be earned by reading the text material, taking the CME examination online at http://www.theclinics.com/home/cme, and completing the evaluation. After taking the test, you will be required to review any and all incorrect answers. Following completion of the test and evaluation, your credit will be awarded and you may print your certificate.

FACULTY DISCLOSURE/CONFLICT OF INTEREST

The University of Virginia School of Medicine, as an ACCME accredited provider, endorses and strives to comply with the Accreditation Council for Continuing Medical Education (ACCME) Standards of Commercial Support, Commonwealth of Virginia statutes, University of Virginia policies and procedures, and associated federal and private regulations and guidelines on the need for disclosure and monitoring of proprietary and financial interests that may affect the scientific integrity and balance of content delivered in continuing medical education activities under our auspices.

The University of Virginia School of Medicine requires that all CME activities accredited through this institution be developed independently and be scientifically rigorous, balanced and objective in the presentation/discussion of its content, theories and practices.

All authors/editors participating in an accredited CME activity are expected to disclose to the readers relevant financial relationships with commercial entities occurring within the past 12 months (such as grants or research support, employee, consultant, stock holder, member of speakers bureau, etc.). The University of Virginia School of Medicine will employ appropriate mechanisms to resolve potential conflicts of interest to maintain the standards of fair and balanced education to the reader. Questions about specific strategies can be directed to the Office of Continuing Medical Education, University of Virginia School of Medicine, Charlottesville, Virginia.

The faculty and staff of the University of Virginia Office of Continuing Medical Education have no financial affiliations to disclose.

The authors/editors listed below have identified no professional/financial affiliations for themselves or their spouse/partner:
Mark Hallet, MD; Davina J. Hensman, MA, MBBS; Joanne Husovski (Acquisitions Editor); LA Massey, MA, MRCP; Fatta B. Nahab, MD; Lubda M. Shah, MD (Test Author); Jan C. M. Zijlmans, MD, PhD; and Ludvic Zrinzo, MD, MSc, FRCSEd (Neuro.Surg).

The authors listed below have identified the following professional/financial affiliations for themselves or their spouse/partner:
Peter G. Bain, MA, MBBS, MD, FRCP is an industry funded research/investigator for Medtronic.
Daniela Berg, MD is an industry funded research/investigator for Janssen Pharmaceutical and TEVA Pharma GmbH, is on the Advisory Committee/Board for Novartis, UCBSchwarzPharma, GSK, and TEVA, and is on the Speakers' Bureau for Novartis, UCBSchwarzPharma, GSK, TEVA, Lundbeck, and Merck.
Jana Godau, MD is on the Speakers' Bureau for UCB and Boehringer.
Andrew J. Lees, MD, FRCP, FMedSci (Guest Editor) is on the Advisory Committee/Board for Novartis, Teva, Meda, Boehringer Ingelheim, GSK, Ipsen, Lundbeck, Allergan, and Orion.
Helen Ling, BMBS, MSc is employed by Reta Lila Weston Institute of Neurological Studies.
A. Peter Moore, MB, ChB, FRCP, MD is an industry funded research/investigator and consultant, and serves on the Advisory Committee/Board and Speakers Bureau, for Ipsen, Allergan, Merz, and Eisai.
Werner Poewe, MD is an industry funded research/investigator and consultant for and serves on the Advisory Committee and Speakers Bureau for BI, GSK, Teva, Novartis, Orion, Astra Zeneca, Schering Plough, and UCB.
Klaus Seppi, MD is on the Speakers' Bureau for UCB, BI, GSK, Novartis, and Lundbeck.
Klaus Tatsch, MD is an industry funded research/investigator for GE Health Care, and serves on the Advisory Committee/Board for Bayer Schering.
Tarek A. Yousry, MD, FRCR (Guest Editor) is an industry funded research/investigator for Biogen Idec, ASK and Novartis.

Disclosure of Discussion of Non-FDA Approved Uses for Pharmaceutical Products and/or Medical Devices.
The University of Virginia School of Medicine, as an ACCME provider, requires that all faculty presenters identify and disclose any off-label uses for pharmaceutical and medical device products. The University of Virginia School of Medicine recommends that each physician fully review all the available data on new products or procedures prior to clinical use.

TO ENROLL

To enroll in the Neuroimaging Clinics of North America Continuing Medical Education program, call customer service at 1-800-654-2452 or sign up online at ***http://www.theclinics.com/home/cme***. The CME program is available to subscribers for an additional annual fee of USD 175.

Neuroimaging Clinics of North America

THE CLINICS ARE NOW AVAILABLE ONLINE!

Access your subscription at:
www.theclinics.com

Contributors

CONSULTING EDITOR

SURESH K. MUKHERJI, MD
Professor and Chief of Neuroradiology and
Head and Neck Radiology; Professor of
Radiology, Otolaryngology Head Neck Surgery
and Radiation Oncology, University of
Michigan Health System, Ann Arbor, Michigan

GUEST EDITORS

TAREK A. YOUSRY, Dr med Habil, FRCR
Lysholm Department of Neuroradiology,
Division of Neuroradiology and Neurophysics,
UCL Institute of Neurology, Queen Square,
London, UK

ANDREW J. LEES, MD, FRCP, FMedSci
Reta Lila Weston Institute of Neurological
Studies, Institute of Neurology, University
College London, UK

AUTHORS

PETER G. BAIN, MA, MBBS, MD, FRCP
Department of Neurosciences, Charing Cross
Hospital, London, United Kingdom

DANIELA BERG, MD
Department of Neurodegeneration, Center
of Neurology and Hertie Institute for Clinical
Brain Research, University of Tübingen,
Tübingen, Germany

JANA GODAU, MD
Department of Neurodegeneration, Center
of Neurology and Hertie Institute for Clinical
Brain Research, University of Tübingen,
Tübingen, Germany

MARK HALLETT, MD
Chief, Human Motor Control Section,
Medical Neurology Branch, National Institute
of Neurological Disorders and Stroke, NIH,
Bethesda, Maryland

DAVINA J. HENSMAN, MA, MBBS
Department of Neurosciences, Charing Cross
Hospital, London, United Kingdom

ANDREW J. LEES, MD, FRCP, FMedSci
Reta Lila Weston Institute of Neurological
Studies, Institute of Neurology, University
College London, London, United Kingdom

HELEN LING, BMBS, MSc
Reta Lila Weston Institute of Neurological
Studies, Institute of Neurology, University
College London, London, United Kingdom

L.A. MASSEY, MA, MRCP
Sara Koe PSP Research Centre,
UCL Institute of Neurology, London,
United Kingdom

A.P. MOORE, MB, ChB, FRCP, MD
Consultant Neurologist, Honorary Senior
Lecturer in Neurology, Liverpool University,
The Walton Centre for Neurology and
Neurosurgery, Lower Lane, Liverpool,
United Kingdom

FATTA B. NAHAB, MD
Assistant Professor of Neurology, University
of Miami Miller School of Medicine, Miami,
Florida

WERNER POEWE, MD
Department of Neurology, Innsbruck Medical University, Anichstrasse, Innsbruck, Austria

KLAUS SEPPI, MD
Department of Neurology, Innsbruck Medical University, Anichstrasse, Innsbruck, Austria

KLAUS TATSCH, MD
Professor of Nuclear Medicine, Department of Nuclear Medicine, Municipal Hospital Karlsruhe Inc., Germany

T.A. YOUSRY, Dr med Habil, FRCR
Professor, Lysholm Department of Neuroradiology, National Hospital for Neurology and Neurosurgery, Queen Square, London, United Kingdom

JAN C.M. ZIJLMANS, MD, PhD
Department of Neurology, Amphia Hospital, Breda, The Netherlands

LUDVIC ZRINZO, MD, MSc, FRCSEd (Neuro.Surg)
Consultant Neurosurgeon, Victor Horsley Department of Neurosurgery, National Hospital for Neurology and Neurosurgery, University College London Hospitals NHS Foundation Trust; Consultant Neurosurgeon & Senior Clinical Researcher, Unit of Functional Neurosurgery, Sobell Department of Motor Neuroscience and Movement Disorders, Institute of Neurology, University College London, London, United Kingdom

Contents

> Classification of diseases aids understanding and activity by creating an overview. No single classification can serve all purposes, and it is helpful to be aware of the range of methods available and to understand what they set out to achieve. This article focuses on factors that help the interaction between clinicians and radiologists, with the aim of clarifying how these schemes are generated.

> The substantia nigra and subthalamic nucleus are two key structures in the midbrain that are very important in movement disorders, particularly those associated with parkinsonism. Using conventional magnetic resonance (MR) imaging, the anatomic description of both these structures can be challenging. This article describes the importance of understanding the underlying anatomy and some of the changes associated with pathology in these structures. Advances in MR imaging are discussed, including high-field MR imaging, diffusion tensor imaging, inversion-recovery imaging, and susceptibility-weighted imaging, with particular reference to the substantia nigra and subthalamic nucleus. Understanding of MR imaging features of these nuclei needs to be firmly based on underlying knowledge of anatomy and pathology from postmortem studies, and more work is needed in this field.

> Parkinson disease (PD) is the most common neurodegenerative cause of parkinsonism, followed by progressive supranuclear palsy and multiple system atrophy (MSA). Despite published consensus operational criteria for the diagnosis of PD and the various atypical parkinsonian disorders (APD) such as progressive supranuclear palsy, Parkinson variant of MSA, and corticobasal degeneration, differentiation of these clinical entities may be challenging, particularly in the early stages of the disease. Diagnosis of PD and its distinction from APD and symptomatic parkinsonism is crucial for the clinical evaluation, as these disorders differ in prognosis, treatment response, and molecular pathogenesis. Despite limitations the different modern magnetic resonance (MR) techniques have undoubtedly added to the differential diagnosis of neurodegenerative parkinsonism. This article focuses on static or structural conventional MR imaging techniques including standard T2-weighted,

T1-weighted, and proton-density sequences, as well as different advanced techniques, including methods to assess regional cerebral atrophy quantitatively such as magnetic resonance volumetry, diffusion tensor and diffusion-weighted imaging, and magnetization transfer imaging, to assist in the differential diagnosis of neurodegenerative parkinsonian disorders.

Extrapyramidal syndromes (ES) belong to the most common neurologic illnesses. Because new and promising therapeutic options are currently under development, there is a substantial demand for molecular imaging procedures with the potential to identify the pathologic changes of those illnesses. This article gives an overview of the current positron emission tomography and single photon emission computed tomography applications for diagnosing ES and focuses on their use in clinical practice.

Parkinsonism is a syndrome that features bradykinesia (slowness of the initiation of voluntary movement) and at least 1 of the following conditions: rest tremor, muscular rigidity, or postural instability. Criteria for the clinical diagnosis of vascular parkinsonism (VP) have been proposed, which are derived from a postmortem examination study. Computed tomography and magnetic resonance imaging can support this clinical diagnosis with positive imaging findings. Dopamine transporter single-photon emission computed tomography may also be of help to distinguish VP from Parkinson disease and other parkinsonisms.

The role for neuroimaging in the management of patients with tremor is gradually increasing, particularly with respect to stereotactic neurosurgery and deep brain stimulation where less than 2-mm tolerance is required for accurate electrode placement. The routine use of single photon emission CT technology to image the nigrostriatal dopaminergic system is proving helpful in distinguishing essential and dystonic tremors from neurodegenerative forms of parkinsonism and in improving our understanding of the pathophysiology of rarer tremors.

Transcranial B-mode sonography (TCS) may provide supplementary information to other neuroimaging methods, adding valuable information to the diagnosis and differential diagnosis of movement disorders. The value of TCS in the differential and early diagnosis of Parkinson disease (PD) has been proven. There is increasing evidence that substantia nigra hyperechogenicity, the ultrasound marker typical for PD, may disclose a nigrostriatal vulnerability if found in healthy people, which may contribute to defining high-risk groups for this neurodegenerative disorder. This article provides information about the ultrasound procedure, its specific diagnostic value, and its limitations. Pathophysiologic mechanisms leading to changes in the reflection of ultrasound waves are discussed.

Dedication

To Indra, for her continuous support; to Lina and Norine, for the joy they give me every day; to my brother, for his companionship; to my mother, for her dedication and everlasting affection; and, of course, to you, my father. All you were to me is in this one word: Father. You prepared me for everything in life, but nothing could have prepared me for this. To your memory.

Your son.
In love and pain.

Tarek A. Yousry

E-mail address:
t.yousry@ion.ucl.ac.uk

Neuroimag Clin N Am 20 (2010) xi
doi:10.1016/j.nic.2009.10.003

Preface

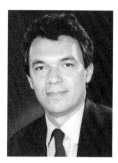
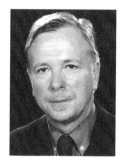

Tarek A. Yousry, Dr med Habil, FRCR   Andrew J. Lees, MD, FRCP, FMedSci
Guest Editors

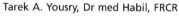

For some time, the main role of neuroimaging in the field of movement disorders was to exclude uncommon but potentially reversible structural abnormalities. However, the advent of magnetic resonance imaging and related techniques, such as diffusion tensor imaging, as well as nuclear medicine techniques, such as positron emission tomography (PET) and dopamine transporter single photon emission computed tomography (SPECT) imaging (DaT-scan), opened up new opportunities to diagnose movement disorders on the basis of objective findings. Nevertheless, the practical value of various neuroimaging techniques in clinical routine is not well known and their potential future development is not well appreciated. With this in mind, we approached leaders in the field who can both assess the relevance of various imaging tools and present their insight into the latest advances from a research perspective. This issue therefore starts by providing an overview of the clinical classification of movement disorders, and then describes the imaging anatomy of some of the structures involved in such disorders. This is followed by an assessment of magnetic resonance and nuclear medicine techniques in various movement disorders. We dedicated an article to the role of transcranial ultrasound, a technique that is gaining a lot of interest and could be of important practical relevance soon. A case-based approach provides real-life scenarios to demonstrate the contribution of neuroimaging techniques to the diagnosis and management of movement disorders. The issue concludes by addressing the important role of imaging in the surgical treatment of these disorders.

We hope readers will find this issue of practical relevance and a stimulus for more in-depth readings in this field.

We are grateful to all the authors who contributed to this issue and we wish to thank the editor of *Neuroimaging Clinics of North America* for encouragement, support, assistance, and patience.

Tarek A. Yousry, Dr med Habil, FRCR
Lysholm Department of Neuroradiology
Division of Neuroradiology and Neurophysics
UCL Institute of Neurology
Queen Square, London, UK

Andrew J. Lees, MD, FRCP, FMedSci
Reta Lila Weston Institute of Neurological
Studies, UCL Institute of Neurology
1 Wakefield Street, London, UK

E-mail addresses:
t.yousry@ion.ucl.ac.uk (T.A. Yousry)
alees@ion.ucl.ac.uk (A.J. Lees)

doi:10.1016/j.nic.2009.10.004

neuroimaging.theclinics.com

Classification of Movement Disorders

A.P. Moore, MB, ChB, FRCP, MD

KEYWORD

• Movement disorder classification

Classification of diseases aids understanding and activity at many levels. It can help to make sense of an otherwise bewildering morass of confusion by creating at least an overview. No single classification can serve all purposes, and it is helpful to be aware of the range of methods available and to understand what they set out to achieve. This article focuses on factors that help the interaction between clinicians and radiologists, with the aim of clarifying how these schemes are generated. Other articles give detailed classifications of the various main movement disorders.

The clinical process starts with the patient and the clinical features presented or uncovered in the history and elicited by examination. If the clinical picture includes a movement disorder, the doctor will probably first attempt to classify it by considering the type or types of movement, will explore the settings in which it occurs or is relieved, and will seek the cause to enable effective treatment. Each stage offers different classifications and subdivisions. Important spin-offs from the classification in individual patients include research, broader management of diseases, and health services, and these too can generate their own schemes.

The movement disorder may constitute the main problem, it may be a feature of a broader disease or its treatment, or be a side issue. As the understanding of diseases changes, it is becoming apparent that a given movement disorder can have different causes. Furthermore, a given underlying disease, even one that seems to be tightly defined, can present with a variety of abnormal movements; simply labeling the clinical phenomena is only a start. Examples include Huntington disease; best known as a cause of chorea, it can present with parkinsonism, especially in younger patients, the

"Westphal variant". 3,4-Dihydrophenylalanine (DOPA)-responsive dystonia is due to well-characterized genetic defects in L-DOPA metabolism. It usually presents in children, with dystonia that classically shows diurnal variation, but can present in later life as DOPA-responsive Parkinsonism instead of dystonia. Combinations of different abnormal movements may add up to a unifying organic diagnosis, as with Parkinson disease (PD) and its classic combination of bradykinesia, rigidity, resting tremor, and postural changes.

PHENOMENOLOGY

Although written descriptions and definitions are helpful and necessary, they are often inadequate and liable to misinterpretation, especially if examination is brief or incomplete and the observer not well versed in movement disorder lore. The individual movements seen in chorea, myoclonus, and tics are similar, and the observer has to clarify the broad pattern and timing to make the distinction. Although disease definitions depend on grouping or the relative proportions of individual movement abnormalities, there is further room for error. Tremor may be declared "dystonic tremor" because there is associated dystonia rather than because of the characteristics of the tremor itself.

Experienced clinicians, even those involved in setting up these definitions, can disagree about the movements shown by individual patients. The presence or prominence of individual features may vary, and abnormalities may come and go completely, such as dyskinesia in PD. Some observations depend on detailed knowledge and understanding of circumstance and the normal, for example a musician's dystonia is easier to detect

Department of Neurology, Liverpool University, The Walton Centre for Neurology and Neurosurgery, Lower Lane, Liverpool L9 7LJ, UK
E-mail address: peter.moore@thewaltoncentre.nhs.uk

Neuroimag Clin N Am 20 (2010) 1–6
doi:10.1016/j.nic.2009.08.018
1052-5149/09/$ – see front matter © 2010 Elsevier Inc. All rights reserved.

and classify if the observer has some knowledge of music. Some components of an abnormal movement may inform or confuse the assessment of others. Is a possibly parkinsonian limb moving slowly because of rigidity, or is there bradykinesia? Other decisions may be influenced by the clinician's interpretation of the cause based on other factors. Could apparent akinesia be due to apraxia?

Video, sound, mechanical, electronic, neurophysiological, or other recordings can aid understanding and classification, especially if the relevant features are too fast, infrequent, or fleeting for accurate observation by the unaided senses. Much interpretation can still be required, and formal blinded comparisons reveal significant rates of inter- and intraobserver disagreement for individual movement abnormalities and for compound diagnoses like Parkinson disease.

Despite all this, experienced clinicians can usually agree on the individual phenomena present, especially if both can examine the patient, or at least discuss him or her and view recordings of the abnormalities.

TYPES OF MOVEMENT

Movements can be willed, automatic, or hybrid, and may be classified as:

- Voluntary: willed and either self-initiated or triggered by an external event.
- Automatic: learned and performed without conscious effort, such as walking.
- Semivoluntary: induced by an internal cue such as itch, discomfort, or an obsession.
- Involuntary: tendon reflexes, physiologic myoclonus, myokymia.

There is a continuum of movement suppressibility. Semivoluntary movements are more often suppressible, at least for a while, and involuntary movements are less often or never suppressible.

TERMINOLOGY AND BOUNDARIES IN MOVEMENT DISORDERS

Clinicians generally reserve the term "movement disorder" for movements driven by somatic muscle, and do not regard most autonomic involuntary activities as a movement disorders. There are a few exceptions, such as palatal myoclonus. Some authorities do not class epilepsy, weakness, or spasticity as movement disorders. The term "abnormal involuntary movements," (AIMs), is often used as an umbrella for movement disorders in general, and particularly the hyperkinetic movements. Despite there being subtle differences, some terms tend to be used interchangeably,

such as bradykinesia (strictly, *slow* movement), hypokinesia (reduced amplitude), akinesia (*no* movement). This example rarely matters diagnostically, especially as there is other no word that readily encompasses the overall concept.

Confusingly, hypokinesia is also used as a generic term for all disorders with not enough movement, whereas bradykinesia and akinesia are generally reserved for the typical slowness of parkinsonism. Dyskinesia blends at its less mobile extreme with dystonia, and is often used to describe the drug-induced dystonic movements seen in Parkinson disease.

Disease "Plus" (eg, PD+ or Dystonia+)

The term "plus" describes disorders with a prominent primary group of features (eg, parkinsonism or dystonia) that are combined with some additional features. Thus parkinsonism plus abnormal eye movements may be due to progressive supranuclear palsy (PSP). These syndromes are extremely helpful in narrowing the range of causes and minimizing the need for "scattergun" investigations. Clinicians usually begin their attempts at classification by focusing on the most prominent features, and considering other problems as add-ons, but it can sometimes be a helpful strategy to invert the process.

Fashions

Diagnoses and classifications are liable to change with time, in part because of linguistic undertones and innuendo. For example, in movement disorders, as in medicine generally, atypical or bizarre features (and even the simple use of those words in a clinical description) may suggest a psychogenic disorder. However, the history of movement disorders is littered with "psychiatric" diseases such as dystonia, which are now recognized as usually organic. This switch reached a point at which labeling a movement "dystonic" was tantamount to deciding it was organic. This has clearly gone too far, as "dystonic" movements can have a nonorganic basis, as can many other movement disorders. It can take considerable expertise to make the distinction.

TYPES OF ABNORMAL MOVEMENT

Abnormal movements are traditionally divided into those involving too much movement (hyperkinesia), or not enough (hypokinesia, bradykinesia or akinesia). Some would add a third category of unnatural movement (dyskinesia), but this is generally a subset of the hyperkinesias. This classification is not entirely logical; for instance, placing spasticity and rigidity in different camps even though there is too much muscle activity in both disorders. Tonic or clonic epilepsy is obviously an abnormal movement, but tends to be dealt with by epileptologists rather than movement disorder specialists.

Intrinsic Clinical Characteristics

Some of these types of abnormal movement are subdivided by their intrinsic characteristics in ways that help the diagnostic process. Thus tremor may be described as intention tremor (by implication cerebellar), resting tremor (parkinsonian), or postural (essential or idiopathic). Associated features may refine the diagnostic label, as when tremor accompanied by dystonia is labeled dystonic tremor. Stiffness is classed as rigidity when it is felt on slow and fast passive movement and in all directions, often with some cogwheeling. It then suggests extrapyramidal disease. Spasticity is increased muscle tone that is sensitive to velocity and often felt more in one direction than the other. It may exhibit the clasp-knife phenomenon, and reflects pyramidal disease.

The anatomic distribution of a movement abnormality such as dystonia or tremor may give etiologic clues. A full breakdown and definitions of all of these subtypes is beyond the scope of this article. Sometimes it is difficult to subclassify, or there may be features of more than 1 subtype, for instance a mixture of postural and resting tremor is increasingly recognized in parkinsonism.

Nonorganic Movement Disorders

Clinicians can sometimes decide between organic and nonorganic movement abnormalities when the movements are sufficiently atypical, but often it is only the associated features that permit the distinction.

Associated Features

Clues related to the history, examination and investigation results, such as the age of onset, time course, genetic or environmental factors, causative or curative drugs, additional movement disorders, or involvement of other neurologic or general medical systems, may all contribute to the classification. Thus Parkinson disease or dystonia presenting in young people is more likely to be genetic. A patient presenting with dementia early in the course of parkinsonism might have Lewy body dementia (LBD), or a patient with dystonia plus liver pathology could have Wilson disease. Dystonia can be highly situation specific, leading to classifications such as the occupational cramps. It may be fairly persistent or may be paroxysmal and triggered by characteristic combinations of metabolic and other stresses.

DIFFERENTIAL DIAGNOSIS: CLASSIFICATIONS
General Clinical Classifications of Movement Disorders

Each of the main movement disorders has several clinical classification schemes, but a frequent approach is to split them broadly into etiologic groups as follows:

○ Primary (idiopathic): the movement disorder is the only feature, and there is no detectable underlying cause or neurodegeneration. The disease-plus syndromes are similar but include some additional clinical features.
○ Secondary or symptomatic, with identifiable causes such as injuries, tumors, infections, stroke, inflammatory or metabolic disease, and drugs.
○ Heredodegenerative diseases
○ Psychogenic

This classification is often only loosely applied, and the categories are not always mutually exclusive, so that some authorities combine primary and heredodegenerative disorders as primary or primary degenerative even if there is a clearly defined genetic cause. For instance, DYT1 dystonia, with its known gene, still exemplifies the primary dystonias in many classifications.

Physiology

The phenomena described in **Box 1** are generally defined in terms of their pathophysiology. Clinicians need to understand the normal physiology of movement to make sense of abnormal movements. In turn, study of the abnormalities may illuminate the normal processes of movement. Physiologic measurements can be used as important features in disease classification. Electromyography can distinguish myotonia from spasticity, or frequency analysis may tell type or subtype of tremor: orthostatic tremor has a characteristic 16-Hz signature, a parkinsonian tremor will be much slower, perhaps 5 Hz. More subtle studies can help identify the anatomic source of myoclonus by showing a consistent sequence of muscle activation as the triggering stimulus passes up or down the spinal cord.

Anatomy

Movement disorders are classically linked to basal ganglia disease, but **Box 1** reveals others originating, at least in part, from most sectors of the nervous system, including cortex (epilepsy,

---

Box 1
Main types of abnormal or involuntary movement

Hypokinesias

Apraxia

Bradykinesia (akinesia/hypokinesia)

Cataplexy

Drop attacks

Epileptic atonias and suspension of activity

Freezing (eg, gait hesitation)

Hypothyroid/hypothermic slowness

Psychiatric slowness (eg, catatonia, depression, obsessional slowness)

Rigidity

Stiff muscles

Thixotropy

Weakness

Hyperkinesias

Akathisia

Alien limb

Ataxia

Ballism

Chorea

Dyskinesia

Dystonia

Epileptic tonic/clonic

Hemifacial spasm

Mirror movements

Myoclonus, including hyperekplexia (startle)

Myokymia

Myorhythmia

Painful feet and moving toes

Punding

Restless legs

Rippling muscles

Shivering

Spasticity

Stereotypy

Synkinesis

Tics

Tonic spasms

Tetany

Tremor

---

apraxia), brain stem (palatal myoclonus, tonic spasms), cerebellum (tremor), cranial nerve (synkinesis, hemifacial spasm), spinal cord (some myoclonus, spasticity, stiff man), peripheral nerve (synkinesis, painful feet with moving toes), neuromuscular junction (weakness), and even from muscle (rippling muscle disease, fibrosis, calcification). Pathology may lie in the sensory system, as in sensory ataxia. Tremor may occur in immunoglobulin-related peripheral neuropathies. The underlying pathology may be mixed or unclear: for instance, it is possible that dystonia has an important sensory component, or even relates primarily to the ability to integrate motor and sensory information. Abnormalities may be found in several systems, making it difficult to know which is primary and which others are downstream consequences or merely bystander effects.

Imaging

Classification of the type of movement disorder often identifies the systems affected and allows focused investigation, including imaging, which may reveal characteristic patterns of change. Equally, there are classifications that depend on imaging findings. In the past, these have usually been purely anatomic, such as lists of causes of basal ganglia calcification, or characteristic patterns of atrophy or high or low magnetic resistance (MR) signals. The advent of functional imaging with single photon emission computed tomography (SPECT), positron emission tomography (PET), functional magnetic resonance imaging (fMRI), magnetoencephalography (MEG) and so forth is generating new classifications. These may merely support anatomic changes seen on more conventional imaging, but they can provide entirely new insights, such as imaging patterns of chemical or ligand receptor characteristics to distinguish idiopathic Parkinson disease from PD+ syndromes or essential tremor. Functional imaging studies are a special form of classification by physiology.

Classification by Pathology, Biochemistry, Genetics, and Immunology

Neurologists have a long history of classifying diseases minutely by their clinical and epidemiologic features, and this habit has meshed well with advances in the more "scientific" disciplines. Tightly defined clinical syndromes provide scientists with groups of patients likely to have something in common. Rapid developments in the basic sciences are in turn causing a steady evolution in disease classifications in ways that have improved understand of the causes of disease, and may lead eventually to class treatments of disorders sharing similar processes.

Pathology of movement disorders
A prime example is the discovery that particular protein aggregations occur in a variety of disorders that were previously considered distinct. Thus corticobasal degeneration (CBD) and PSP are tauopathies with accumulation of tau protein, whereas idiopathic Parkinson disease, LBD and multiple system atrophy (MSA) are α-synucleinopathies. The differing clinical presentations of apparently the same pathologic process reflect the anatomic patterns of distribution of affected cells. Myoclonus, extrapyramidal, pyramidal, dyspraxic, and other movement disorders may occur in prion diseases.

These new associations are being linked by discoveries of many different genetic defects in the processes of synthesis or degradation of the relevant proteins. Defects at various points along the pathways can have unpredictably similar or different clinical and pathologic effects.

Biochemistry of movement disorders
The field of movement disorders is dominated by Parkinson disease, in which the key defining abnormality is partly biochemical, with loss of dopaminergic function in the basal ganglia. This discovery opened up much broader exploration of dopamine and other neurotransmitter functions, and new classifications of movement and psychiatric disorders based on their biochemical features. Other groupings of disease include those with chemical accumulation or deficiency states. Brain iron accumulation occurs in Hallervorden-Spatz disease (also known as *pantothenate kinase-associated neurodegeneration* [PKAN]), aceruloplasminaemia, neuroferritinopathy and other diseases, and copper accumulation occurs in Wilson disease. Thiamine or vitamin E deficiency leads to eye movement abnormalities and cerebellar disease, respectively. Many of the childhood- or adult-onset metabolic disorders cause movement disorders, among other problems, and many of the biochemical diseases turn out to have a genetic basis.

Genetics of movement disorders
Early genetic studies of some major movement disorders used classical epidemiologic techniques such as twin studies, but sometimes provided confusing results, as in parkinsonism. Some of these broad syndromes encompass many different genetic defects, often interacting with external environmental factors such as chemicals (drugs, industrial, or agricultural toxins) or infections, or internal disorders (tumors, autoimmune disease).

There are expanding lists of movement disorders within classes of nuclear or nonnuclear genetic abnormality, such as the trinucleotide repeat disorders like Huntington disease and fragile X tremor-ataxia syndrome (FXTAS), or with single gene deletions, perhaps causing gain of function or loss of function. Some mitochondrial genome disorders generate abnormal movements, typically myoclonus, parkinsonism, or ataxia.

Immunology of movement disorders
Many movement disorders are linked to autoimmunity, with antibodies generated against tissues involved in movement or movement control. Sometimes these act through broader brain damage that includes movement-related structures, as when antiphospholipid antibodies lead to stroke, or with aquaporin 4 antibodies causing myelopathy. There is an increasing recognition of antibodies that directly target the organs of movement, such as anti–basal ganglia antibodies after streptococcal disease (one of a group labeled pediatric autoimmune neuropsychiatric disorders associated with streptococcal infections [PANDAS]), and perhaps following influenza (encephalitis lethargica). Other anatomic targets include particular cells in the cortex, cerebellum, or spinal cord, and physiologic targets including ion and ligand channels in the central and peripheral nervous systems. These antibodies are often paraneoplastic. The archetypal neurologic immunologic disease, myasthenia gravis, produces a movement abnormality, weakness.

FUTURE BENEFITS FROM CLASSIFICATION

Diagnostic and therapeutic strategies can exploit these new classifications and the associations they provide between diseases. Successful classifications can group or split diseases in new ways that facilitate the development of methods that help in several members of a group.

For example, just as imaging techniques have been developed that reflect dopamine-related functions or iron accumulation, ways to image prion or tau aggregates, for instance, can also be sought.

Classifying a disorder as autoimmune already allows us to deploy immune-based preventive and therapeutic treatments such as steroids, intravenous immunoglobulin (IVIg), plasma exchange, interferons, and other immune suppressants. Alternatively, we can seek out and treat any neoplasm to directly remove the source of antibodies.

Whole classes of treatments now target neural ligand or ion channel receptors. Dopamine agonists or blockers have been helpful treatments in a variety of disorders. Deficiency or accumulation disorders may respond to measures correcting the deficit or surplus. Likewise, treatments that reduce tau production or improve its breakdown, interfere with self-aggregating proteins such as prions, or more generally influence protein degradation pathways, or techniques that repair or circumvent genetic disorders (eg, by blocking trinucleotide repeats) could prove effective for many disorders.

FURTHER READINGS

Fahn S, Jankovic J, Hallett M, et al. Principles and practice of movement disorders. Churchill Livingstone; 2007.

Warner T, Bressman SB. Clinical diagnosis and management of dystonia. Informa Healthcare; 2007.

Anatomy of the Substantia Nigra and Subthalamic Nucleus on MR Imaging

L.A. Massey, MA, MRCP[a], T.A. Yousry, Dr med Habil, FRCR[b],*

KEYWORDS

- Magnetic resonance imaging • Substantia nigra
- Subthalamic nucleus • Parkinsonism

Conventional magnetic resonance (cMR) imaging, including T1-weighted (T1-w), T2-weighted (T2-w) and proton-density–weighted (PD-w) images (often now in combination with fluid-attenuated inversion-recovery (FLAIR) and sometimes, T2*-weighted [T2*-w] imaging) often form the basis of standard MR imaging protocols when investigating movement disorders. Of patients with the hypokinetic-/akinetic-rigid movement disorders, those with Parkinson disease (PD) are by far the largest group, and currently, there are no significant abnormalities detected on cMR imaging. The role of cMR imaging is supportive and may be helpful in excluding structural abnormalities or normal pressure hydrocephalus, for example, in addition to aiding in the planning of stereotactic neurosurgery.

IMPORTANCE OF ANATOMIC ACCURACY ON MR IMAGING

The substantia nigra (SN) and subthalamic nucleus (STN) are key nuclei in PD and parkinsonian illnesses, such as progressive supranuclear palsy (PSP); the SN is severely affected in both conditions but with slightly different topography; the STN is a preferred target in stereotactic surgical techniques in PD (deep-brain stimulation [DBS]) and as a characteristic site of severe pathologic involvement in PSP. These structures and their

components are often difficult to identify on cMR imaging, despite the efforts of many investigators since the 1980s, when MR imaging started to become clinically available. The recent literature has highlighted the importance of anatomic accuracy and shed some light on methods by which this may be improved. Discussion of this literature on the anatomy of the SN and STN on MR imaging will form the substance of this review and a framework for considering an approach to other small brainstem nuclei which are of increasing interest — for esample the pendunculopontine tegmental nucleus (PPN) and locus coeruleus (LC). With improvements in MR imaging technology, including higher field strength and use of diffusion tensor imaging (DTI) and susceptibility-weighted imaging (SWI), there should soon be a far greater ability to visualize these small nuclei during life. This ability should enable accurate anatomic identification of small subcortical nuclei, enhance the ability to make early diagnoses, and monitor progression of the natural history and treatment effects.

IRON AND CONVENTIONAL MR IMAGING

Using cMR imaging, brain morphology and signal intensity can be assessed. Normal change associated with increasing age is an important consideration—changes in signal intensity on T2-w MR

[a] Sara Koe PSP Research Centre, Department of Molecular Neuroscience, UCL Institute of Neurology, 1 Wakefield Street, London, WC1N 1PJ, UK
[b] Lysholm Department of neurology and neurosurgery NHNN, UCL Institute of neurology, Queen Square, London, WC1N 3BG, UK
* Corresponding author.
E-mail address: t.yousry@ion.ucl.ac.uk (T.A. Yousry).

Neuroimag Clin N Am 20 (2010) 7–27
doi:10.1016/j.nic.2009.10.001

imaging reflecting, largely, the deposition of iron. In the normal human brain, iron is deposited symmetrically in the globus pallidus (GP), red nucleus (RN), SN, putamen, and dentate and caudate nuclei.[1] In animals (monkeys), iron is also deposited in the striato-pallido-nigral and cerebellar corticonuclear systems.[2] Iron is also deposited in the STN.[3]

T2-w MR images at 1.5T show T2-w signal hypointensity in the GP, SN pars reticulata (SNr), RN, dentate, putamen, and subcortical U fibers[4] and also hypointensity within the STN.[5,6] These hypointense regions correlate at least partially, but not perfectly, with the distribution of iron seen on Perl stain (see later discussion)[7] (Fig. 1).

On T2-w MR imaging at 1.5T, deep gray matter nuclei are not hypointense at birth and iron is deposited sequentially in the GP, RN, SN, and dentate nuclei.[8] By the age of 25 years, these structures are all hypointense relative to cortical gray matter. During normal adult life, the pallidum becomes progressively more hypointense but the RN, SN, and dentate remain unchanged. Changes with age in the STN are not well studied.

IRON IN DISEASE

Iron deposition is increased in the SN in PD, PSP, and multiple system atrophy (MSA).[9–11] Iron is deposited with ferritin and also binds strongly to neuromelanin[12]; it is found deposited in brainstem Lewy bodies (the pathologic hallmark of PD).[13] Most iron detected is present in ferric Fe^{3+} form bound to ferritin,[14] and in PD, iron is deposited leading to increased loading of ferritin.[15] Little is known about iron deposition in the STN, although it does seem to be present in control postmortem tissue,[3,7] and there is some indirect evidence that iron deposition is increased in the STN in PD.[16] The role of iron deposition in the pathogenesis of

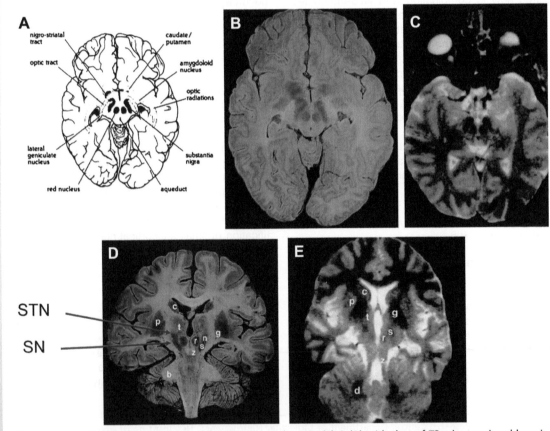

Fig. 1. Comparison of the distribution of iron using Perl's stain (B) & (D) with that of T2w image signal hypointensity (C) & (E). In the axial images (B) & (C) hypointensity and intense Perl stain can be seen in the RN and SN. In the coronal images (D) and (E) the STN is also seen on the Perl stain (D) – upper and outer region of intense staining which has been called the *Suderoku sign* on MRI.[112] c caudate; p putamen; t thalamus; r red nucleus; s substantia nigra; n subthalamic nucleus; z brachium conjurictivum; b brachium pontis; d dentate nucleus. (*From* Rutledge JN, Hilal SK, et al. Study of movement disorders and brain iron by MR. AJR Am J Roentgenol 1987;149(2):365–79; with permission.)

neurodegenerative disease is still unclear; Zecca et al[14] provide a review of iron in ageing and neurodegeneration.

A NOTE ON ANATOMIC TERMS

The use of anatomic terms in the radiological and pathologic literature is slightly different: radiologists prefer the terms anterior, posterior, superior, and inferior, which may be referred to as ventral, dorsal, rostral, and caudal in the anatomic/histologic literature (Table 1). In the region of the STN, this is more confusing because dorsal and superior may be synonymous, and indeed, this is discussed more in the section on the STN anatomy.[17] In the following discussion, the terms anterior, posterior, superior, and inferior have been used for consistency and ease of reference.

SN
The Anatomy of the SN

Location, orientation and constituent parts
The substantia nigra (SN) is found in the mesencephalon posterior (dorsal) to the crus cerebri, anterior (ventral) to the midbrain tegmentum, and just inferior to the red nucleus. It runs from the level of the mamillary nuclei down the ventral pontine nuclei.[18] It lies inferior and lateral to the RN and takes up an oblique angle, being most lateral at its superior boundary. It is divided into 2 anatomically and functionally distinct parts: the inferior (caudal) and posterior (dorsal) SN pars compacta (SNc) containing melanized neurons, and the superior (rostral) and anterior (ventral) SNr.

Connections
The neurons of the pars compacta project to the striatum using the neurotransmitter dopamine—"the nigrostriatal pathway"—and there is a reciprocal projection from the striatum that uses (GABA), substance P, and dynorphin—"the striatonigral pathway." The neurons of the SNr form one of the output nuclei of the basal ganglia along with the internal segment of the GP; they project to the thalamus using the neurotransmitter GABA.[19]

Table 1
Interchangeable anatomic terms applied to the midbrain

Anatomic	Radiological
Ventral	Anterior
Dorsal	Posterior
Rostral	Superior
Caudal	Inferior

Internal anatomy
The anatomy of the SN is complex and various schemes have been proposed for the internal anatomy of neurons within it.[20–26] Olzewski and Baxter[25] described 3 tiers of melanized neurons in the posterior-anterior (dorsoventral) axis (alpha, beta and gamma). The gamma group of pigmented neurons are called the SN pars dorsalis by Damier and colleagues[26]; however, the use of substance P to delineate the anatomy of the SN based on the striatonigral innervation excludes this group, which is labeled the parabrachial pigmented nucleus and separates the SN and RN; Halliday[27] provides a review of the SN anatomy (Fig. 2). Within the SNc itself, Fearnley and Lees[22] identified 2 tiers of pigmented neurons, the posterior and anterior (dorsal and ventral) tiers. These are orientated in an anteromedial block along the course of the mesencephalon. The anterior and posterior tiers can be further subdivided by anatomic location (splitting the 2 tiers into 3 subdivisions) or by using calbindin immunohistochemistry, which stains the neuropil but reveals discrete calbindin-poor zones called nigrosomes where pigmented neurons reside.[26] The SNc also contains medial and lateral clusters of pigmented neurons (pars medialis and pars lateralis).

Pathology in the SN

Macroscopic pallor of the usually darkly stained SNc is visible to the naked eye in PD (SN literally meaning "black substance"); Fig. 2A shows the normal macroscopic appearance. Loss of pigmented neurons at the rate of 4.7% per decade is found in normal aging, and in PD, 45% of pigmented neurons are lost in the first decade of the disease.[22] Importantly, neuronal loss is not homogenous throughout the SN—in normal aging, the most severely affected region is the medial anterior and posterior tiers; in PD, the loss is greatest in the lateral anterior tier (ventrolateral tier).[22,24] The progression of pathology in PD seems to move from the inferior anterolateral SNc and progress superiorly, medially, and posteriorly.[28] Other neurodegenerative conditions show increased loss with different topography: the posterior tier in MSA and posteromedial tier in PSP.[22] In PSP, the SNc is affected and there is loss of up to 70% of SNr neurons.[29] In MSA, the SNc is more affected in MSA-P (parkinsonism type, striatonigral degeneration) than MSA-C (cerebellar type, olivopontocerebellar atrophy).[30]

MR Imaging of the SN

Conventional MR imaging
Early MR imaging studies compared iron distribution as defined by Perl stain with reduced signal

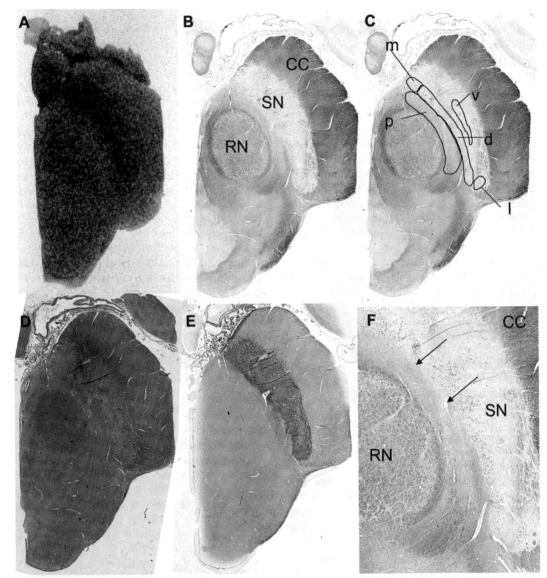

Fig. 2. The histology of the SN. (*A*) macroscopic image showing the dark staining of neuromelanin. (*B*) Luxol fast blue stain of the SN showing white matter as blue. (*C*) Clusters of pigmented neurons within the SN showing the pars medialis (m), pars lateralis (l), and the dorsal (d) and ventral (v) tiers. The parabrachial pigmented nucleus (p) is outlined. In PD, the ventral and lateral tiers are more severely affected.[22] (*D*) Perl stain showing the distribution of iron within the SN. (*E*) Substance P immunohistochemistry showing the extent of the SN. (*F*) The pigmented cells within the SN and the myelinated fibers lying in the region between the RN and SN in a ventrodorsal orientation (*arrows*). (*Photography courtesy of* Susan Stoneham, Queen Square Brain Bank for Neurologic Disorders; histologic stains *courtesy of* Kate Strand, Queen Square Brain Bank for Neurologic Disorders).

intensity (hypointensity) on T2-w MR imaging.[4,7,31–33] The match was felt to be "precise",[31] with reduction in T2-w signal intensity and reduced T2 relaxation time in regions of most intense Perl staining.[4] Based on signal intensity, a medial region of signal hypointensity in the midbrain was attributed to the SNr and the lateral region with higher signal intensity, to the SNc.[31] Furthermore, "smudging" of the SNr was seen in atypical parkinsonism,[31] and "restoration" of the T2-w signal intensity, in the lateral SN in PD.[7] Further studies found the correlation of Perl staining and T2-w signal hypointensity to be imperfect in other anatomic locations, with less T2-w signal hypointensity in the putamen and caudate and more hypointensity in the internal capsule, commissures, and corpus callosum than would be expected from Perl studies (see **Fig. 1**).[7]

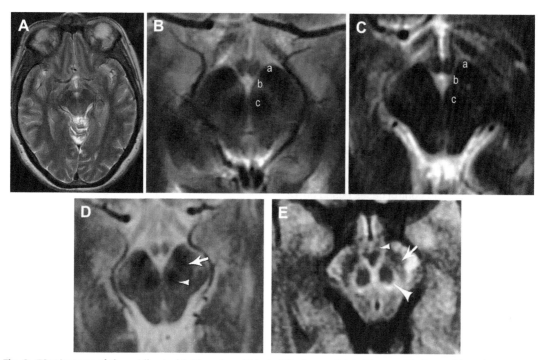

Fig. 3. T2w images of the midbrain (*A–D*) and mulitshot diffusion weighted image (*E*). Control (*A&B*): a cerebral peduncle, b substantia nigra, c red nucleus; (*C*) PD with loss of clarity of margins of structures. (*D*) and (*E*) are T2w and Diffusion weighted images respectively showing the contrast in SN outline. (*D*) *Arrow* SN, *arrow head* RN; [E] *small arrow head* mammillary body, *large arrow* substantia nigra ((*D*) and (*E*)). (Images (*D*) and (*E*) *from* Adachi M, Hosoya T, Haku T, et al. Evaluation of the substantia nigra in patients with Parkinsonian syndrome accomplished using multishot diffusion-weighted MR imaging. AJNR Am J Neuroradiol 1999;20(8):1500–6; with permission; other images *courtesy of* Dr Mario Miranda, Division of Radiology, Department of Medicine, School of Medicine, University of Panama, Panama City, Panama.)

To clarify the situation, comparison of MR characteristics and histology in the same tissue should be instructive. However, imaging postmortem tissue to date has not significantly improved our understanding of the origin of the signal from the SN. At 2T (repetition time [TR] 800 ms, echo time [TE] 40 ms, 8 excitations) and at 1.5T (TR 500 ms, TE 25, 2 excitations), the SN was identified as a broad band of relatively bright signal between the tegmental and tectal structures.[34,35] In a further comparison of histologic sections and post mortem T2-w MR images, the SN is seen as a poorly defined high-signal structure in the midbrain anterior to the relatively hypointense cerebral peduncles.[36]

Using iron to define anatomy and in disease

Using T2-w images to define the anatomy of the SN,[37] it has been proposed that the SNc is represented by a region of high signal intensity, between the low signal intensity of the RN and that of the SNr in the anterior-posterior axis (see Fig. 3). This fits with the known distribution of iron in the RN and SNr and therefore has become

the basis for the description of abnormalities seen in disease (see **Fig.** 2D).

Reduced width of the SNc in PD was attributed to an increase in iron deposition in the SNr and/or loss of dopaminergic melanized neurons in the SNc.[37] Subsequent studies also showed reduction in SNc width[38–41] or described a smudging of the SNr hypointensity with reduction in the distance between the RN and the SNr in PD and also in other parkinsonian syndromes.[32,42–44] Other abnormalities described in PD (and atypical parkinsonian illnesses, MSA and PSP) include T2-w signal hyperintensity within the SNr[38] or restoration of normal signal intensity in the lateral SN (ie, loss of the hypointense signal).[7,39] However, only one study has found a correlation between the width of the SNc and a measure of clinical severity.[40]

MR relaxometry in the SN

If iron is the chief determinant of the MR imaging hypointensity on T2-w imaging and is also deposited during disease, measuring the T2 relaxation time may provide insight into the progression of disease. Indeed, the literature contains many attempts to use T2 relaxometry measurements as surrogate markers of disease. However, T2 measurements alone are not reliable enough; this is borne out by the fact that T2 measurements in the SN overlap in control and PD groups,[45] and T2 measurements are affected by local iron-induced field inhomogeneities and the differing magnetic susceptibilities of tissue interfaces, thus reflecting global field inhomogeneities.[46]

Using a gradient recalled-echo sequence to measure T2 and T2* at 3T, it is possible to discriminate between PD and control cases based on T2' (a component of T2* that is a more specific measure of tissue iron) and R_2' (1/T2').[46] Additionally, R_2' measurements correlate with simple motor scores in PD, implying a relationship between clinical features, iron deposition in the SN, and R_2'.[47] This is also found using the partially refocused interleaved multiple echo (PRIME) MRI sequence to measure R_2^* and R_2' relaxation rates, which are higher in the SN of PD than in controls at 1.5T.[48]

The role of field strength and novel iron-sensitive techniques

Field strength is a crucial consideration, because relaxation rates theoretically increase (inversely as relaxation times fall) with magnetic field strength and the concentration of iron. Measurement of iron/ferritin specifically using field-dependent R_2 increase (FDRI) at 0.5T and 1.5T showed an increase in FDRI in SNc and SNr in addition to other regions (GP, putamen, caudate nucleus, and frontal white matter) in patients with PD younger than 60 years. Later-onset patients had decreased FDRI compared with age-matched controls, which may have been because of reduced iron/ferritin and increased free iron deposition, although the influence of age-related changes in iron deposition should also be considered.[49]

Later, novel iron contrast sequences were used at 4T showing asymmetrical differences in the SN in PD, and quantitative differences in PD from controls attributed to iron deposition (using $T_{2\rho}$) and neuronal loss (using $T_{1\rho}$) in the SN; these changes were seen despite no significant changes in T2 being observed.[50]

In addition, the regional predilection of PD for the anterolateral SNc has been studied using multiple gradient-echo MR imaging at 3T to measure R_2^* in a paradigm designed to minimize magnetic field inhomogeneities arising from tissue-tissue and air-tissue interfaces; regional increase in iron content as evidenced by increased R_2^* in the lateral SNc was found in early untreated PD, which correlated with United Parkinson Disease Rating Scale scores.[51]

Defining the anatomy of the SN on MR imaging

Ever since the original description of the anatomy of the SN on MRI,[37] there has been concern about the accuracy of the anatomic correlation.[44,47,51,52] The description of the high-signal band on T2-w images corresponding to the SNc has been questioned. Immunohistochemical techniques suggest that the SNc does not extend all the way to the RN and that pigmented neurons in this location are part of the parabrachial pigmented nucleus.[27] There are also white matter tracts in this region, and rather than representing the SN, the hyperintense T2-w band could be the site of white matter of the nigrostriatal tracts.[18,47,52] Furthermore, signal changes attributed to the SN using different MR imaging modalities appear to have different precise anatomic origins (see later discussion).

PD-w and fast short inversion time inversion-recovery imaging

PD-w and fast short inversion time inversion-recovery (FSTIR) enhance gray matter-white matter contrast thereby reducing the effect of "iron-related" mechanisms of T2-w imaging. The SN appears as a tilted bandlike structure of hyperintense gray matter, without discriminating between the SNc and SNr (**Fig. 4**).[53] On coronal images, the SN is seen inferolaterally to the RN, and on sagittal images, anteroinferiorly. This is in line with anatomic descriptions of the SN and is different in location to that of the hypointense regions seen on T2-w images, which has been attributed to the SNr. Comparison of FSTIR with Perl stain shows that the hypointense region overlaps only with the most superior and anterior portion of the SN (**Fig. 5**).[53]

Segmented inversion-recovery imaging

Heavily T1-w inversion-recovery images show signal abnormalities in the SN in PD at 1.5T. On so-called gray-matter suppressed (GMS) inversion-recovery sequences, there is increased signal in areas of degeneration; on white-matter suppressed (WMS) sequences, the signal is reduced in the same regions.[54] Using a ratio of inversion-recovery acquisitions, WMS to GMS, the sensitivity of the signal changes is increased. A gradient of increasing signal abnormality from medial to lateral and inferior is found in PD.[22,54,55] A radiological index of the lateral and medial SN signal correlates with clinical severity.[55] Using the WMS image to define the boundaries, an automatic segmentation technique can be applied to extract the SN (called segmented inversion-recovery imaging [SIRRIM]).[56] In PSP, a reverse gradient is

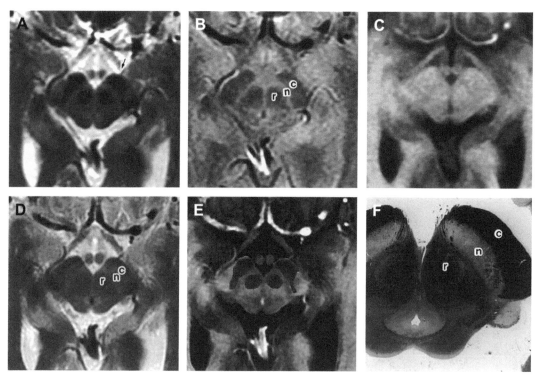

Fig. 4. Comparison of axial midbrain images at 1.5T. (*A*) T2w. (*B*) PDw. (*C*) T1w. (*D*) fast STIR. (*E*) Video-inverted fast STIR with T2w hypointense regions superimposed. (*F*) axial cadaveric specimen image. r RN; n SN; c cerebral peduncle. (*From* Oikawa H, Sasaki M, Tamakawa Y, et al. The substantia nigra in Parkinson disease: proton density-weighted spin-echo and fast short inversion time inversion-recovery MR findings. AJNR Am J Neuroradiol 2002;23(10):1747–56; with permission.)

seen, with the most severe changes being medial, and the known atrophy of the SN can be visualized (**Fig. 6**). SIRRIM could potentially distinguish PD from healthy controls and from essential tremor, PSP, and MSA and may be potentially sensitive enough to assess changes in the early course of the disease.[57] However, in other studies, this technique was not as robust as ^{18}F-Dopa PET in distinguishing control from PD[58] or parkinsonism (PD or parkin mutation-positive parkinsonism), with 67% of parkin mutation-positive patients, 44% of PD patients, and 25% of controls identified as abnormal. However, more generalized signal changes are seen in patients with parkin mutation who have more widespread nigral pathology, which may in part be because of the longer disease duration of parkin patients.[59] Although there are clearly technical problems to overcome, including aspects of acquisition and processing (eg, division versus subtraction of GMS and WMS images), and problems with artefactual appearances, high variance in data, and the issue of field strength, abnormalities when present reflect the pathologic topography.[57,59,60] Further nonsubjective quantitative analysis of the spectra from the SN using SIRRIM, the spin-lattice

distribution index, may be more accurate and less user-dependent, but further studies are needed.[61] Three-dimensional techniques of acquisition of GMS and WMS data enable accurate segmentation of the SN using the driven-equilibrium single-pulse observation of T1 acquisition.[62]

Imaging neuromelanin

Melanin has been shown to increase longitudinal T1 relaxation rates in vitro,[63] and thus, the LC and SN on T1-w fast spin-echo (FSE) images at 3T may appear hyperintense. At 3T, the combination of increased spatial resolution, the doubling of the signal-to-noise ratio (SNR), and the prolonging of T1 relaxation times in combination with FSE-related off-resonance magnetization transfer effects suppressing brain tissue signal all contribute toward this finding. The location of the T1-w hyperintense signal matches the distribution of melanized neurons in the SNc and LC in control postmortem tissue.[64] In PD, the hyperintense signal is lost as expected. This approach can be used to visualize age-dependent changes in the LC.[65] The role of iron in the SNc may mask the effect of prolonging T1 via susceptibility effects;

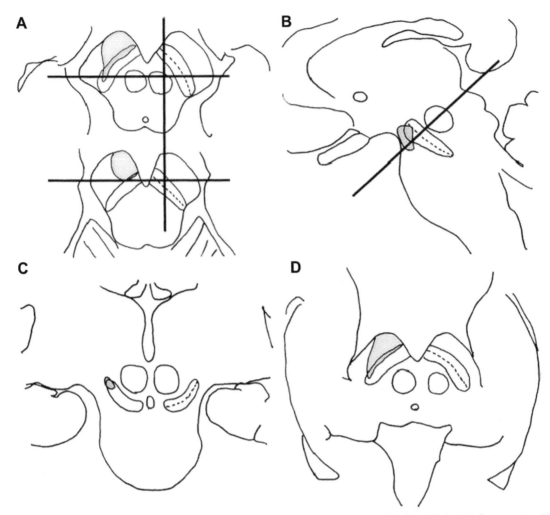

Fig. 5. Comparison of the position of hypointense signal on T2-w images with that of the SN from anatomic atlases in the axial (*A*), sagittal (*B*), coronal (*C*), and oblique coronal plane (*D*). (*From* Oikawa H, Sasaki M, Tamakawa Y, et al. The substantia nigra in Parkinson disease: proton density-weighted spin-echo and fast short inversion time inversion-recovery MR findings. AJNR Am J Neuroradiol 2002;23(10):1747–56; with permission.)

this may explain why the changes in the SNc are less remarkable than in the LC.[64]

Diffusion-weighted imaging
The boundaries of the SN may be more accurately seen by assessing the structures immediately surrounding the SN, rather than the signal from the SN itself. The orientation of white matter tracts in the midbrain makes them a useful marker of the SN borders; using multishot diffusion-weighted images, the outline of the SN is clearly visualized. The SN is represented by a crescent of low signal intensity situated between the higher signal of the tegmentum of the midbrain and the cerebral peduncle (see **Fig.** 1C, D).[52] The SN is most clearly seen when the orientation of the diffusion gradient was in the left-right direction, perpendicular to the pyramidal tracts (superior-inferior) and those between the SN and RN that are orientated anterior-posterior (see **Fig.** 2F). When the width of the SN is measured in PD, it is within the normal range, but secondary parkinsonism is associated with SN atrophy. This is in line with pathologic studies where atrophy of the SN is not prominent in PD.

The importance of understanding the pathologic topography is illustrated in the recent literature. Early quantitative MRI measurements within the whole SN showed no significant difference in regional apparent diffusion coefficient (rADC) in PD, MSA-P, and PSP.[66,67] Later, a significant reduction in fractional anisotropy (FA) and nonsignificant increase in ADC were found in a medial SN

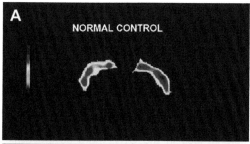

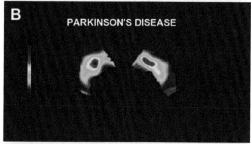

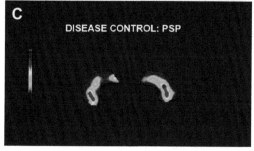

Fig. 6. Axial images of the SN using SIRRIM. Loss of signal is seen ventrolaterally in PD and medially in PSP. (*From* Hutchinson M, Raff U, Lebedev S. MRI correlates of pathology in parkinsonism: segmented inversion-recovery ratio imaging (SIRRIM). Neuroimage 2003;20(3):1899–02; with permission.)

region of interest in PD, which correlated inversely with clinical severity, although the separation was not great enough to enable this technique to be used as a diagnostic marker.[68] However, using high-resolution DTI at 3T, the most lateral SN region of interest had significantly lower FA in early (<2 years) untreated PD and enabled discrimination from an unaffected cohort with 100% sensitivity and specificity.[69] Reduced FA along the path of the nigrostriatal projection is evident, particularly in regions of interest near the SN in PD.[70] Furthermore, FA loss is observed along the nigrostriatal projection in PD and PSP, and in among other regions, the STN, GP, and cortex in PSP, as would be expected from the pathology.

Magnetization transfer imaging

Magnetization transfer imaging (MTI) relies on the transfer of energy between protons bound in macromolecules, such as myelin, and those in mobile molecules, such as water. Changes correlate with myelin and axonal density, and as such, MTI enables good contrast between gray and white matter. The SN can be clearly seen as a region of relatively increased signal in comparison with the cerebral peduncles and RN on magnetization transfer saturated images.[71,72] MTI has been proposed recently as a more reliable technique than T1-w images, which are conventionally used for segmentation of subcortical gray matter structures. This is particularly important as the SN is not well-defined on T1-w images.[72]

STN
Anatomy of the STN

Location, composition and orientation
The STN was first described by Luys in 1865, but the clinical significance of this structure was not obvious until the description of hemiballism arising from a vascular lesion in the region of the STN.[73] The STN contains approximately 550, 000 projection neurons in humans.[74,75] It lies in the mesencephalon and is an almond-shaped structure; the internal capsule is on its anterolateral border and the fields of Forel and hypothalamus (with which the borders are blurred) on its medial border, with the SN ventrally (inferior and lateral), and the zona incerta (ZI) and lenticular fasciculus dorsally (superior and medial) positioned.[19,76,77] It is obliquely orientated with regard to standard anatomic axes being 20° oblique to the horizontal plane, 35% oblique to the sagittal plane, and 55° oblique to the frontal plane.[76] Its dimensions are approximately $3 \times 5 \times 12$ mm in humans.[78]

Connections
From its medial border runs the subthalamic fasciculus to the pallidum across the internal capsule. Projections from the pallidum (ansa lenticularis and lenticular fasciculus) encase the STN after their passage through the internal capsule and on their way to the thalamus, before joining with the fibers from the RN and brainstem to become the thalamic fasciculus.[18,19,77] Afferent connections to the STN come from the cortex (glutamate), the external segment of the GP (GABA), the thalamus (glutamate), the SNc (dopamine), the PPN and laterodorsal tegmental nucleus (acetyl choline, glutamate), the dorsal raphe nuclei (serotonin), and other nuclei. The main efferent projections (glutamate) are to the internal and external segments of the GP, the SNc and SNr, the striatum and brainstem nuclei, including the PPN, and the anterior (ventral) tegmental area.[79,80] The projections maintain topography and are complex single neurons projecting to

more than one of the basal ganglia output structures.[79–81]

Internal anatomy

The STN can be divided into 3 sections determined by its connectivity: the dorsolateral portion forms part of the sensorimotor circuit; the ventromedial portion, the associative circuit; and the medial portion, the limbic circuit.[79,82–84]

The STN lies in the mesencephalon at the junction of the rostral Meynert brainstem axis and more caudal Forel brainstem axis, which lie at an angle of approximately 90° to 105° to each other.[17] This has led to some confusion about the use of the terms dorsal and ventral and some have proposed that the sensorimotor STN, which has been ascribed the anatomic label of "dorsolateral," should be referred to as the anterior, lateral, and superior STN, suggesting that superior may be less ambiguous than dorsal in the context of STN anatomy.

Iron in the STN

Along with other structures in the basal ganglia, iron is known to be deposited in the STN (Fig. 7, also see Fig. 1). Although not commented on, this is clearly visible in the article by Rutledge and colleagues.[7] However, there is no published data on how this changes with age or disease,[3] although there is some indirect evidence of increased iron deposition in the STN in PD.[16]

Pathology in the STN

The STN is a key structure in the surgical treatment of PD, being a target for subthalamotomy and DBS.[85,86] However, in PD itself, there is little pathologic change.[75] Dopamine depletion leads to pathophysiological changes in the STN, first demonstrated in animal models of parkinsonism.[87–92] This was the stimulus for considering the STN as a surgical target in PD in humans.[85,93] In contrast, the STN is a key structure pathologically in PSP.[75,94,95] It is also involved in other conditions, such as postencephalitic parkinsonism and corticobasal degeneration.[96,97] In PSP, there is significant volume loss, and 45% to 85% neuronal loss in the STN, more severe clinical phenotypes associated with more severe involvement of the STN.[75,94,95]

MRI of the STN

Conventional MR imaging

The STN is seen as a region of T-2w hypointensity, anterior and lateral to the RN lying at a slightly oblique angle in the axial plane (Fig. 8). However, the SN also gives rise to a hypointense signal, and the border between the STN and SN is not clearly seen on axial T2-w images.[17] In the coronal plane, the anatomy is somewhat clearer because the SN lies inferior and medial to the STN.

The difficulties in accurate identification have led to the development of several techniques to guide the placement of electrodes targeted to the STN. The surgical target is based on the Schaltenbrand and Wahren atlas coordinates. These are based on the anterior commissure (AC)-posterior commissure (PC) line and the midcommissural point (MCP). The STN is usually located 12 mm lateral to the midline, 2 mm behind the MCP, and 4 mm ventral to the AC-PC plane.[98] The small size of the STN, its oblique orientation, the almond or lens shape, and considerable intra- and interindividual variation in anatomy contribute to the difficulties in targeting this structure during surgical

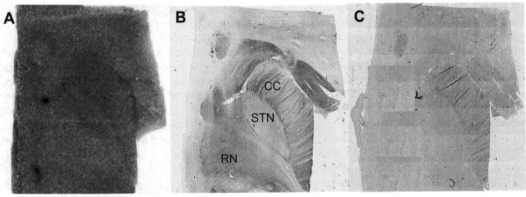

Fig. 7. Histological images of the STN (center of images). (A) macroscopic image. (B) Luxol Fast Blue stains white matter tracts blue. (C) Perl stain for iron which is seen within the STN[3] and in the pallidofugal tracts crossing the internal capsule. RN red nucleus; STN subthalamic nucleus; CC crus cerebri. (*Photography courtesy of* Susan Stoneham, Queen Square Brain Bank for Neurologic Disorders; histologic and Perl stains *courtesy of* Kate Strand, Queen Square Brain Bank for Neurologic Disorders).

procedures. Consequently, confirmation of electrode placement is sought, using techniques including clinical assessment, microelectrode recordings,[99,100] or local field potentials.[101] Some target the STN directly, on the basis that it can be clearly and reliably identified pre- and postoperatively using T2-w MR imaging,[6] although others suggest that the STN cannot be visualized reliably.[102] However, in a study on a patient who died soon after having STN electrodes placed using electophysiological techniques[103,104] and despite good clinical efficacy immediately postoperatively, the electrode position was outside the medial border of the STN and not within the dorsolateral sensorimotor portion of the STN. Further work indicates that clinical efficacy alone is not a reliable indicator of lead position when compared with postmortem study.[105]

Location and anatomy of the STN on MR imaging

The anatomic correlate of the low signal on T2-w images has not been extensively studied to date. Early MR publications indicate that there may be iron in the STN, which is responsible for the lower T2-w signal intensity[7]; however, later studies speculate that the lower signal may be related to high neuronal density rather than iron per se.[100] A detailed study compared the hypointense appearance of the STN on T2-w images obtained from patients with PD, with the Schaltenbrand and Wahren atlas digitally registered to the same images (Fig. 9). In a separate autopsy control case, the distribution of iron using Perl stain was also registered to the Schaltenbrand and Wahren atlas. The anterior half of the STN as defined by the Schaltenbrand and Wahren atlas was always hypointense on T2-w images, whereas the posterior portions were less reliably so.[3] Similarly, Perl stain showed iron deposition in the anteromedial half of the STN more prominently than in the posterolateral pole. By comparison with animal studies that show the dorsolateral STN being the sensorimotor portion and hence the supposed preferred neurosurgical target, this would imply that the associative territory of the STN has relatively more iron deposition and is thus more visible on T2-w MR imaging than the dorsolateral sensorimotor portion.

Variability in the position and dimensions of the STN

The Schaltenbrand and Wahren atlas is the most commonly used reference for indirect planning of STN electrode placement.[98] This atlas was based on fixed pathologic specimens from only 4 controls of different ages. A postmortem study has shown that the coordinates of the center of

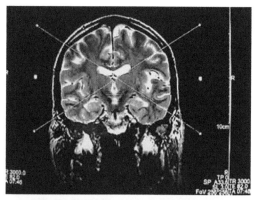

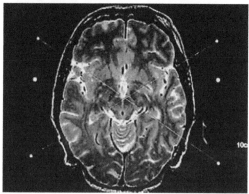

Fig. 8. 1.5T T-2w coronal (*upper image*) and axial (*lower image*) MR images showing a T2-w hypointense structure lateral and dorsal to the red nuclei which is in the region of the STN. (*From* Hariz MI, Krack P, Melvill R, et al. A quick and universal method for stereotactic visualization of the subthalamic nucleus before and after implantation of deep brain stimulation electrodes. Stereotact Funct Neurosurg 2003;80(1–4):96–101; with permission.)

the STN change between the ages of 29 and 84 with respect to the AC-PC line (the standard reference)[106]: the center of the STN moves 3.9 mm cranially, 2.6 mm laterally, and 0.2 mm anteriorly. Additionally, there is a change in shape, the nucleus becoming wider in the mediolateral plane but smaller in the superior-inferior and anterior-posterior planes.

The interindividual variation in position of the STN is evident from studying the location of an atlas-derived STN target and direct imaging of the STN[107]; the directly visualized target was on average 1.7 mm medial, 0.7 mm anterior, and 0.7 mm ventral to the atlas-derived target. Further evidence of the interindividual variability comes from other work showing differences in size, orientation, and target coordinates between direct and indirect methods[108,109] and comparing T2-w images of the STN with the Talairach and Schaltenbrand atlases.[110]

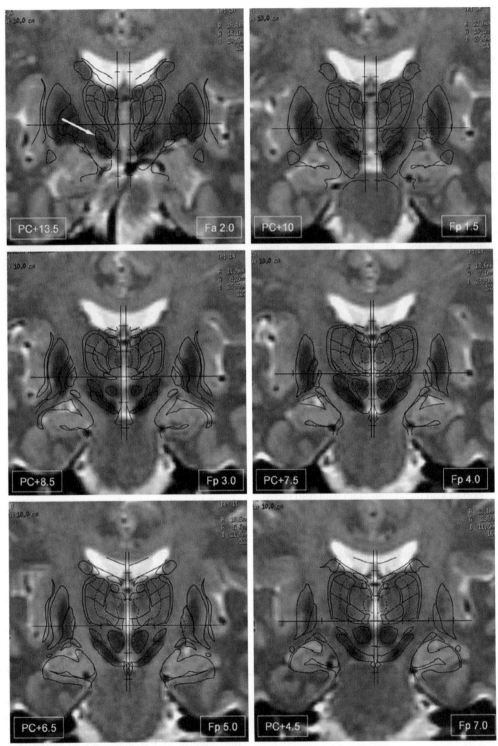

Fig. 9. Coronal T2w images fused with the Schaltenbrand and Wahren atlas moving from anterior to posterior [figures indicate location with respect to the PC in mm]. STN arrowed in first image. Note that the STN region is most hypointense anteriorly and least hypointense posteriorly. (*From* Dormont D, Ricciardi KG, Tande D, et al. Is the subthalamic nucleus hypointense on T2-weighted images? A correlation study using MR imaging and stereotactic atlas data. AJNR Am J Neuroradiol 2004;25(9):1516–23; with permission.)

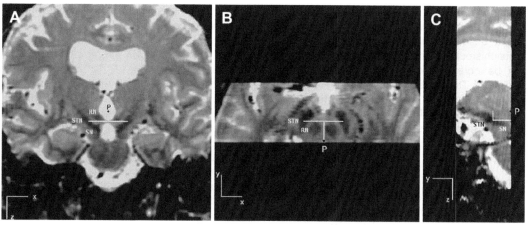

Fig. 10. (A) Coronal, (B) axial and (C) sagittal views of the STN using T2-w MR imaging. The position of the STN in relation to the SN, RN, and projection of the AC-PC line (P) can be seen, with particular reference to the RN. (*From* Bejjani BP, Dormont D, Pidoux B, et al. Bilateral subthalamic stimulation for Parkinson's disease by using three-dimensional stereotactic magnetic resonance imaging and electrophysiological guidance. J Neurosurg 2000;92(4):615–25; with permission.)

Locating the STN and using internal landmarks

T2-w images currently provide the most readily available direct visualization of the STN. However, problems with image resolution and distortion due to susceptibility effects place limitations on the utility of direct targeting using T2-w images.[102] Distortion of the STN anatomy can be up to 2.19 mm in the frequency-encoding direction and 3.81 mm in the slice selection.[111] As a result of this, fusion of T2-w and T1-w images is often used to reduce the effect of distortion and improve anatomic accuracy.

The identification of anatomic structures can be supported and facilitated by using defined landmarks. These landmarks can be direct or indirect. Direct landmarks take advantage of specific features of the structure to be identified. One such landmark is the "Sukeroku sign"; in the coronal plane, in a section perpendicular to the AC-PC line, and at the level of the internal auditory canal, the STN appears like Sukeroku's makeup just lateral to his eye.[112] Another landmark is the "dent internal capsule sign"; in the axial plane, the STN can be seen more medially as a dent in the internal capsule outline.[112]

Indirect landmarks take advantage of specific, easily identifiable features of a structure that have a defined relationship with the structure to be identified:

The RN

- In the axial plane the anterior border of the RN corresponds to the midpoint of the STN, and the coordinates of the STN can be calculated with reference to the projection of the AC-PC line in 3 dimensions using multiplanar reformatted T2-w images (**Fig. 10**).[5]
- A point 3 mm lateral to the most lateral border of the RN and 2 mm inferior to the most superior border was 3.19 mm from the optimal DBS contact[113]

The supramammillary commissure on T1-w imaging is posterior to the optic tracts and mammillary bodies and is one of the few structures connecting the right- and left-sided nuclei.[102] The top of the midportion of the thickest central portion of the supramammillary commissure is 4 mm below the AC-PC line at the same level as the STN, which is found 12 mm directly lateral to this point.[102]

The mammillary body and the posterior commissure

- Using 9.4T MR imaging of postmortem tissue, a line connecting the mammillary body and the posterior commissure lies in the same plane as the STN and may be useful in targeting the STN along the rostro-caudal axis of the midbrain.[114]

The Mammillothalamic tract is clearly identifiable on axial images and is 5 to 6 mm medial to the anterior border of the STN.

A composite targeting method using the postmammillary commissure, the mammillothalamic tract, the RN, and the T2-w hypointensity in the anterior part of the STN has also been shown to be accurate to within 3.19 mm of the final optimal electrode contact location.[115]

Another approach has focused on the construction of a 3-dimensional atlas of the human basal ganglia based on histologic stains (Nissl) and immunohistochemistry for calbindin, which can then be coregistered to T1-w and T2-w MR imaging.[116] This atlas can then be registered to individual patient MR images for accurate identification of the STN with a less than 1-mm discrepancy from electrophysiological signatures.[117]

High-field MR imaging

The increasing availability of high-field 3T MR imaging has many advantages, including increased susceptibility effect of iron, improvements in SNRs, and shorter acquisition times. The main drawbacks relate to safety concerns in patients with metal implants.

At 3T, MR imaging enables clear definition of the STN anatomically on T2-w FSE images in a short time, and reduces the need for multiple tract detailed physiologic definition; in one study, the electrophysiological location of the STN was confirmed on the first pass in each case, reducing the operation time and the theoretical risk of hemorrhage (**Fig. 11**).[118] Comparison of FSE T2-w images and FSTIR images at 3T reveals that the STN is well defined in all but its inferior/ventral boundary with the SN on T2-w images; however, FSTIR images enable distinction from the SN as there is a significant difference in signal intensity between the SN and STN using FSTIR.[119] Other studies have shown that improvements in the SNR and susceptibility contrasts improve spatial resolution of deep brain structures using field strengths of 4.7T[120] and 8T.[121] Indeed, postmortem studies of anatomic tissue specimens at up to 9.4T reveal that it is possible to visualize the microanatomy of the STN and its environs, including many of the local fiber tracts

(**Fig. 12**).[114] This is a promising field as higher-field systems become more widely available.

Recent advances in MR imaging of the STN

Multiple gradient-echo T2* T2* is more sensitive to microscopic susceptibility-induced field gradient effects than T2 and has the advantage of lower radiofrequency exposure via gradient-echo over standard FSE sequences used to obtain T2 images.[122] Using multigradient-echo fast low-angle shot (FLASH) sequence, a combination of T1-w and T2*-w images can be acquired that are of high resolution and inherently coregistered. The former can be used for stereotactic planning and the latter for visualization of iron-related contrast from the STN, which is greater for T2* than T2.[123] Alternatively, a postprocessing method can be used in which multiple intensity-corrected T2*-w images are optimized for iron-rich structures, such as the STN, in compensation for regions of high signal loss due to susceptibility-induced field gradients.[122] This is possible in short acquisition times (under 4 minutes).[122] However, the influence of artifacts related to stereotactic frames, and the electrodes postoperatively, and any potential problems arising from coregistration are still to be addressed.[122,123] Furthermore, the dimensions of small subcortical structures may well be distorted using T2*-w images.[121]

SWI An additional MR contrast mechanism can be obtained using phase images acquired during SWI acquisitions, such as a 3D velocity compensated gradient-echo sequence. Theoretically, iron within structures, such as the STN, accelerates the magnitude of signal-intensity decay because of T2* shortening and increases the resonance frequency, with spins accumulating a phase effect.[124] Phase images contain information about local static field variations, geometry-induced field variations, and local tissue susceptibility.

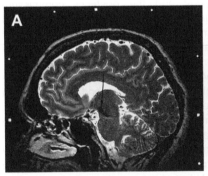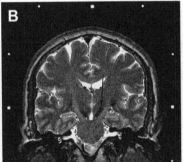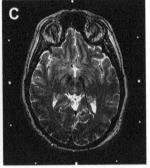

Fig. 11. High field MRI of the STN. (*A–C*) show sagittal, coronal and axial images of the brain during life at 3T. STN arrowed in black. (*From* Slavin KV, Thulborn KR, Wess C, et al. Direct visualization of the human subthalamic nucleus with 3T MR imaging. AJNR Am J Neuroradiol 2006;27(1):80–4; with permission.)

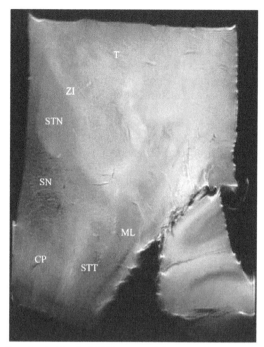

Fig. 12. 9.4 Tesla MRI image of the STN showing the STN in its 'microenvironment' in the sagittal plane in a post-mortem tissue block. T Thalamus; ZI zona Incerta; STN subthalamic nucleus; SN substantia nigra; CP cerebral peduncle; STT spinothalmic tract; ML medial lemniscus. (*From* Rijkers K, Temel Y, Visser-Vandewalle V, et al. The microanatomical environment of the subthalamic nucleus. Technical note. J Neurosurg 2007;107(1):198–201; with permission.)

Postprocessing techniques enable separation of the phase image from the magnitude data; a single SWI acquisition can provide T2* maps of signal intensity magnitude, phase images, and a combination of the two, which is sometimes called the "venogram" because of the high-resolution images of vessels containing deoxyhaemoglobin.[124,125] SWI at 4T clarifies some of the anatomy when compared with lower-field images (1.5T), enabling separation of the STN from the SN in the coronal plane.[125] It has been shown that phase images at high resolution (after zero-filling, the voxel size in this study was 0.45×0.45×0.75 mm) depict the STN more clearly than T2* or combined "venogram" images. Optimization of significant parameters shows that an echo time of 21.6 ms and an acceleration factor of 1.36 for partial parallel encoding using sensitivity encoding enables accurate definition of the STN with a short acquisition time of less than 2.5 minutes.[124] This allowed a reliable separation of the STN from the SN in the axial plane.

Fast gray matter acquisition T1 inversion-recovery Fast gray matter acquisition T1

inversion-recovery (FGATIR) has been developed from T1-w magnetization-prepared rapid acquisition gradient-echo sequences with the aim of nullifying the signal from cerebrospinal fluid and fat.[126] The resulting images are based on signal from gray matter only and this has enabled excellent delineation of gray matter structures surrounded by white matter tracts (eg, the thalamus and GP internus). The STN appears as a hypointense region similar to that seen on STIR, possibly because of the relatively high level of myelination within the STN when compared with surrounding structures[119]: A distinct boundary is seen between the STN and SNr with a contrast-to-noise ratio of 6.06 using FGATIR versus 1.76 on 3D T2-w FLAIR images.[126] Near the superior border of the STN is a high signal region on the FGATIR, the origin of which is not clear, but it may represent either the superior STN or lower ZI.[126] This 3D technique has advantages over the standard T2-w images of the STN in that it is fast, the voxels are near-isotropic, thereby allowing 3D reconstructions, and the resolution is not limited by technical factors but by signal-to-noise and time constraints.

Imaging the STN in PSP
Changes in the STN are remarkable for the paucity of significant findings in a search of the literature, given its importance in conditions such as PSP. However, this is most probably because of technical limitations of imaging such a small structure and its controversial MR imaging anatomy. Nonetheless, volumetric imaging of the midbrain using voxel-based morphometry has shown selective reduction in gray and white matter in the region of the STN within the midbrain in PSP.[127] A reduction in FA in PSP in the subthalamic structures, including the STN, has also been reported.[70]

DTI AND TRACTOGRAPHY

It would be remiss not to discuss DTI and its application in tractography, although, thus far, application of this technique to the brainstem has been restricted to relatively large white matter fiber tracts, such as the cerebellar peduncles, pyramidal tracts, and medial lemniscus.[128–131] Smaller tracts of interest, including the nigrostriatal tract, have not thus far been visible.[132] Using current techniques, there are limitations, including spatial resolution (current best voxel size is 2×2×2, with resulting problems identifying small white matter tracts), signal loss in the brainstem near the STN and SN due to iron-related susceptibility, motion artifacts, crossing fibers within voxels, low SNRs, which increases the duration of imaging required to obtain sufficient SNR, and distortion associated with high-field DTI acquisition. Nonetheless, the topography of cortical and subcortical connections within the STN and PPN using DTI at 3T reveals white matter tract connectivity that corresponds to animal and postmortem human work.[133–135] Also, based on the connectivity of the thalamus, it has been possible to segment the thalamus and derive a probabilistic gray matter parcellation based on the cortical connectivity of the subnuclei.[136,137] The potential of DTI to increase understanding of the anatomy in the brainstem and to help understand the functional relationship of small brainstem nuclei is still unfulfilled.

SUMMARY

To maximize the return on the advances in the technology of MRI, a good grounding in anatomy and pathology is crucial. Direct comparison of imaging and histologic findings has only been performed in a few studies. The relevance of this approach has been demonstrated by recent studies on the SN and STN comparing the distribution of iron with low signal intensity on T2-w images.[3,53] Particularly in the SN, the assumed MR anatomy from early studies has continued to be used for many years despite evident concern about its validity.[44,47,52] Both these regions require intense study with careful pathologic correlation in health and disease.

However, it is possible to visualize small nuclei, including the STN, using conventional techniques in a clinically useful way. The STN can thus be identified using direct and indirect landmarks making it accessible to direct targeting. Even smaller nuclei may be visible using conventional techniques[138] and studies optimizing the image contrast of these structures using currently available techniques will prove fruitful.

With improvements in spatial resolution and SNR at higher field strength, smaller structures, such as the STN, are more clearly visualized.[118] In combination with techniques, such as diffusion-weighted imaging, magnetization transfer imaging, and inversion-recovery imaging, monitoring of these diseases will be an important area of research in the coming years. New methods for assessing iron and the susceptibility effects associated with this are also significant in this regard. Combinations of these techniques in a multimodal assessment and diagnostic algorithm may be useful to assess these diseases with disseminated, yet topographically characteristic, pathology.

ACKNOWLEDGMENTS

Luke Massey is supported by a grant from the PSP Association (UK). The authors are grateful to Mario Miranda for some of the images, and to Susan Stoneham, Catherine Strand, and Professor Tamas Revesz at the Queen Square Brain Bank for Neurologic Disorders for the histologic and pathologic images. This work was undertaken at University College London Hospitals (UCLH)/UCL who received a proportion of funding from the UK Department of Health's National Institute for Health Research Biomedical Research Centers funding scheme (UCLH/UCL Comprehensive Biomedical Research Trust).

REFERENCES

1. Schenck JF, Zimmerman EA. High-field magnetic resonance imaging of brain iron: birth of a biomarker? NMR Biomed 2004;17(7):433–45.
2. Francois C, Nguyen-Legros J, Percheron G. Topographical and cytological localization of iron in rat and monkey brains. Brain Res 1981;215(1–2):317–22.
3. Dormont D, Ricciardi KG, Tande D, et al. Is the subthalamic nucleus hypointense on T2-weighted images? A correlation study using MR imaging and stereotactic atlas data. AJNR Am J Neuroradiol 2004;25(9):1516–23.
4. Drayer B, Burger P, Darwin R, et al. MRI of brain iron. AJR Am J Roentgenol 1986;147(1):103–10.
5. Bejjani BP, Dormont D, Pidoux B, et al. Bilateral subthalamic stimulation for Parkinson's disease by using three-dimensional stereotactic magnetic resonance imaging and electrophysiological guidance. J Neurosurg 2000;92(4):615–25.
6. Hariz MI, Krack P, Melvill R, et al. A quick and universal method for stereotactic visualization of the subthalamic nucleus before and after implantation of deep brain stimulation electrodes. Stereotact Funct Neurosurg 2003;80(1–4):96–101.
7. Rutledge JN, Hilal SK, Silver AJ, et al. Study of movement disorders and brain iron by MR. AJR Am J Roentgenol 1987;149(2):365–79.
8. Aoki S, Okada Y, Nishimura K, et al. Normal deposition of brain iron in childhood and adolescence: MR imaging at 1.5 T. Radiology 1989;172(2):381–5.
9. Dexter DT, Carayon A, Javoy-Agid F, et al. Alterations in the levels of iron, ferritin and other trace metals in Parkinson's disease and other neurodegenerative diseases affecting the basal ganglia. Brain 1991;114(Pt 4):1953–75.
10. Dexter DT, Jenner P, Schapira AH, et al. Alterations in levels of iron, ferritin, and other trace metals in neurodegenerative diseases affecting the basal ganglia. The Royal Kings and Queens Parkinson's

Disease Research Group. Ann Neurol 1992; 32(Suppl):S94–100.

11. Dexter DT, Wells FR, Lees AJ, et al. Increased nigral iron content and alterations in other metal ions occurring in brain in Parkinson's disease. J Neurochem 1989;52(6):1830–6.

12. Jellinger K, Kienzl E, Rumpelmair G, et al. Iron-melanin complex in substantia nigra of parkinsonian brains: an x-ray microanalysis. J Neurochem 1992;59(3):1168–71.

13. Castellani RJ, Siedlak SL, Perry G, et al. Sequestration of iron by Lewy bodies in Parkinson's disease. Acta Neuropathol 2000;100(2):111–4.

14. Zecca L, Youdim MB, Riederer P, et al. Iron, brain ageing and neurodegenerative disorders. Nat Rev Neurosci 2004;5(11):863–73.

15. Griffiths PD, Dobson BR, Jones GR, et al. Iron in the basal ganglia in Parkinson's disease. An in vitro study using extended X-ray absorption fine structure and cryo-electron microscopy. Brain 1999; 122(Pt 4):667–73.

16. Kosta P, Argyropoulou MI, Markoula S, et al. MRI evaluation of the basal ganglia size and iron content in patients with Parkinson's disease. J Neurol 2006;253(1):26–32.

17. Coenen VA, Prescher A, Schmidt T, et al. What is dorso-lateral in the subthalamic Nucleus (STN)?– a topographic and anatomical consideration on the ambiguous description of today's primary target for deep brain stimulation (DBS) surgery. Acta Neurochir (Wien) 2008;150(11):1163–5 [discussion: 1165].

18. Carpenter M, Sutin J. Human neuroanatomy. 8th edition. Baltimore (MD): Williams & Wilkins; 1983.

19. Nieuwenhuys R, Voogd J, van Huijzen C. The Human central nervous system: a synopsis and atlas. 4th revised edition. New York: Springer; 2007.

20. Hassler R. [Zur Pathologie der Paralysis agitans und des Postenzephalitischen Parkinsonismus]. J Psychol Neurol 1938;48:387–476 [in German].

21. German DC, Manaye K, Smith WK, et al. Midbrain dopaminergic cell loss in Parkinson's disease: computer visualization. Ann Neurol 1989;26(4): 507–14.

22. Fearnley JM, Lees AJ. Ageing and Parkinson's disease: substantia nigra regional selectivity. Brain 1991;114(Pt 5):2283–301.

23. Gibb WR, Lees AJ. Anatomy, pigmentation, ventral and dorsal subpopulations of the substantia nigra, and differential cell death in Parkinson's disease. J Neurol Neurosurg Psychiatr 1991;54(5):388–96.

24. Gibb WR. Melanin, tyrosine hydroxylase, calbindin and substance P in the human midbrain and substantia nigra in relation to nigrostriatal projections and differential neuronal susceptibility in Parkinson's disease. Brain Res 1992;581(2):283–91.

25. Olzewski J, Baxter D. Cytoarchitecture of the human brain stem. 2nd edition. Basel: Karger; 1982.

26. Damier P, Hirsch EC, Agid Y, et al. The substantia nigra of the human brain. I. Nigrosomes and the nigral matrix, a compartmental organization based on calbindin D(28K) immunohistochemistry. Brain 1999;122(Pt 8):1421–36.

27. Halliday GM. Substantia nigra and locus coeruleus. Chapter 14. In: Paxinos G, Mai JK, editors. The human nervous system. 2nd edition. Elsevier Academic Press; 2004. p. 451–61.

28. Damier P, Hirsch EC, Agid Y, et al. The substantia nigra of the human brain. II. Patterns of loss of dopamine-containing neurons in Parkinson's disease. Brain 1999;122(Pt 8):1437–48.

29. Hardman CD, Halliday GM, McRitchie DA, et al. Progressive supranuclear palsy affects both the substantia nigra pars compacta and reticulata. Exp Neurol 1997;144(1):183–92.

30. Ozawa T, Paviour D, Quinn NP, et al. The spectrum of pathological involvement of the striatonigral and olivopontocerebellar systems in multiple system atrophy: clinicopathological correlations. Brain 2004;127(Pt 12):2657–71.

31. Drayer BP, Olanow W, Burger P, et al. Parkinson plus syndrome: diagnosis using high field MR imaging of brain iron. Radiology 1986;159(2):493–8.

32. Drayer BP. Imaging of the aging brain. Part II. Pathologic conditions. Radiology 1988;166(3):797–806.

33. Drayer BP. Imaging of the aging brain. Part I. Normal findings. Radiology 1988;166(3):785–96.

34. Solsberg MD, Fournier D, Potts DG. MR imaging of the excised human brainstem: a correlative neuroanatomic study. AJNR Am J Neuroradiol 1990; 11(5):1003–13.

35. Hirsch WL, Kemp SS, Martinez AJ, et al. Anatomy of the brainstem: correlation of in vitro MR images with histologic sections. AJNR Am J Neuroradiol 1989;10(5):923–8.

36. Flannigan BD, Bradley WG Jr, Mazziotta JC, et al. Magnetic resonance imaging of the brainstem: normal structure and basic functional anatomy. Radiology 1985;154(2):375–83.

37. Duguid JR, De La Paz R, DeGroot J. Magnetic resonance imaging of the midbrain in Parkinson's disease. Ann Neurol 1986;20(6):744–7.

38. Braffman BH, Grossman RI, Goldberg HI, et al. MR imaging of Parkinson disease with spin-echo and gradient-echo sequences. AJR Am J Roentgenol 1989;152(1):159–65.

39. Stern MB, Braffman BH, Skolnick BE, et al. Magnetic resonance imaging in Parkinson's disease and parkinsonian syndromes. Neurology 1989;39(11):1524–6.

40. Pujol J, Junque C, Vendrell P, et al. Reduction of the substantia nigra width and motor decline in aging

and Parkinson's disease. Arch Neurol 1992;49(11): 1119–22.

41. Yagishita A, Oda M. Progressive supranuclear palsy: MRI and pathological findings. Neuroradiology 1996;38(Suppl 1):S60–6.

42. Savoiardo M, Strada L, Girotti F, et al. MR imaging in progressive supranuclear palsy and Shy-Drager syndrome. J Comput Assist Tomogr 1989;13(4): 555–60.

43. Savoiardo M, Strada L, Girotti F, et al. Olivopontocerebellar atrophy: MR diagnosis and relationship to multisystem atrophy. Radiology 1990;174(3 Pt 1): 693–6.

44. Savoiardo M, Girotti F, Strada L, et al. Magnetic resonance imaging in progressive supranuclear palsy and other parkinsonian disorders. J Neural Transm Suppl 1994;42:93–110.

45. Antonini A, Leenders KL, Meier D, et al. T2 relaxation time in patients with Parkinson's disease. Neurology 1993;43(4):697–700.

46. Ordidge RJ, Gorell JM, Deniau JC, et al. Assessment of relative brain iron concentrations using T2-weighted and T2*-weighted MRI at 3 Tesla. Magn Reson Med 1994;32(3):335–41.

47. Gorell JM, Ordidge RJ, Brown GG, et al. Increased iron-related MRI contrast in the substantia nigra in Parkinson's disease. Neurology 1995;45(6): 1138–43.

48. Graham JM, Paley MN, Grunewald RA, et al. Brain iron deposition in Parkinson's disease imaged using the PRIME magnetic resonance sequence. Brain 2000;123(Pt 12):2423–31.

49. Bartzokis G, Cummings JL, Markham CH, et al. MRI evaluation of brain iron in earlier- and later-onset Parkinson's disease and normal subjects. Magn Reson Imaging 1999;17(2):213–22.

50. Michaeli S, Oz G, Sorce DJ, et al. Assessment of brain iron and neuronal integrity in patients with Parkinson's disease using novel MRI contrasts. Mov Disord 2007;22(3):334–40.

51. Martin WR, Wieler M, Gee M. Midbrain iron content in early Parkinson disease: a potential biomarker of disease status. Neurology 2008;70(16 Pt 2):1411–7.

52. Adachi M, Hosoya T, Haku T, et al. Evaluation of the substantia nigra in patients with Parkinsonian syndrome accomplished using multishot diffusion-weighted MR imaging. AJNR Am J Neuroradiol 1999;20(8):1500–6.

53. Oikawa H, Sasaki M, Tamakawa Y, et al. The substantia nigra in Parkinson disease: proton density-weighted spin-echo and fast short inversion time inversion-recovery MR findings. AJNR Am J Neuroradiol 2002;23(10):1747–56.

54. Hutchinson M, Raff U. Parkinson's disease: a novel MRI method for determining structural changes in the substantia nigra. J Neurol Neurosurg Psychiatr 1999;67(6):815–8.

55. Hutchinson M, Raff U. Structural changes of the substantia nigra in Parkinson's disease as revealed by MR imaging. AJNR Am J Neuroradiol 2000; 21(4):697–701.

56. Hutchinson M, Raff U, Lebedev S. MRI correlates of pathology in parkinsonism: segmented inversion recovery ratio imaging (SIRRIM). Neuroimage 2003;20(3):1899–902.

57. Raff U, Hutchinson M, Rojas GM, et al. Inversion recovery MRI in idiopathic Parkinson disease is a very sensitive tool to assess neurodegeneration in the substantia nigra: preliminary investigation. Acad Radiol 2006;13(6):721–7.

58. Hu MT, White SJ, Herlihy AH, et al. A comparison of (18)F-dopa PET and inversion recovery MRI in the diagnosis of Parkinson's disease. Neurology 2001;56(9):1195–200.

59. Hu MT, Scherfler C, Khan NL, et al. Nigral degeneration and striatal dopaminergic dysfunction in idiopathic and Parkin-linked Parkinson's disease. Mov Disord 2006;21(3):299–305.

60. Minati L, Grisoli M, Carella F, et al. Imaging degeneration of the substantia nigra in Parkinson disease with inversion-recovery MR imaging. AJNR Am J Neuroradiol 2007;28(2): 309–13.

61. Hutchinson M, Raff U. Detection of Parkinson's disease by MRI: spin-lattice distribution imaging. Mov Disord 2008;23(14):1991–7.

62. Menke RA, Scholz J, Miller KL, et al. MRI characteristics of the substantia nigra in Parkinson's disease: a combined quantitative T1 and DTI study. Neuroimage 2009;47(2):435–41.

63. Enochs WS, Hyslop WB, Bennett HF, et al. Sources of the increased longitudinal relaxation rates observed in melanotic melanoma. An in vitro study of synthetic melanins. Invest Radiol 1989;24(10): 794–804.

64. Sasaki M, Shibata E, Tohyama K, et al. Neuromelanin magnetic resonance imaging of locus ceruleus and substantia nigra in Parkinson's disease. Neuroreport 2006;17(11):1215–8.

65. Shibata E, Sasaki M, Tohyama K, et al. Age-related changes in locus ceruleus on neuromelanin magnetic resonance imaging at 3 Tesla. Magn Reson Med Sci 2006;5(4):197–200.

66. Schocke MF, Seppi K, Esterhammer R, et al. Diffusion-weighted MRI differentiates the Parkinson variant of multiple system atrophy from PD. Neurology 2002;58(4):575–80.

67. Seppi K, Schocke MF, Esterhammer R, et al. Diffusion-weighted imaging discriminates progressive supranuclear palsy from PD, but not from the parkinson variant of multiple system atrophy. Neurology 2003;60(6):922–7.

68. Chan LL, Rumpel H, Yap K, et al. Case control study of diffusion tensor imaging in Parkinson's

disease. J Neurol Neurosurg Psychiatr 2007; 78(12):1383–6.

69. Vaillancourt DE, Spraker MB, Prodoehl J, et al. High-resolution diffusion tensor imaging in the substantia nigra of de novo Parkinson disease. Neurology 2009;72(16):1378–84.

70. Yoshikawa K, Nakata Y, Yamada K, et al. Early pathological changes in the parkinsonian brain demonstrated by diffusion tensor MRI. J Neurol Neurosurg Psychiatr 2004;75(3):481–4.

71. Eckert T, Sailer M, Kaufmann J, et al. Differentiation of idiopathic Parkinson's disease, multiple system atrophy, progressive supranuclear palsy, and healthy controls using magnetization transfer imaging. Neuroimage 2004;21(1):229–35.

72. Helms G, Draganski B, Frackowiak R, et al. Improved segmentation of deep brain grey matter structures using magnetization transfer (MT) parameter maps. Neuroimage 2009;47(1):194–8.

73. Purdon Martin J. Hemichorea resulting from a local lesion of the brain. (The syndrome of the body of Luys). Brain 1927;50:637–51.

74. Rafols JA, Fox CA. The neurons in the primate subthalamic nucleus: a Golgi and electron microscopic study. J Comp Neurol 1976;168(1):75–111.

75. Hardman CD, Halliday GM, McRitchie DA, et al. The subthalamic nucleus in Parkinson's disease and progressive supranuclear palsy. J Neuropathol Exp Neurol 1997;56(2):132–42.

76. Yelnik J, Percheron G. Subthalamic neurons in primates: a quantitative and comparative analysis. Neuroscience 1979;4(11):1717–43.

77. Hamani C, Saint-Cyr JA, Fraser J, et al. The subthalamic nucleus in the context of movement disorders. Brain 2004;127(Pt 1):4–20.

78. Yelnik J. Functional anatomy of the basal ganglia. Mov Disord 2002;17(Suppl 3):S15–21.

79. Parent A, Hazrati LN. Functional anatomy of the basal ganglia. II. The place of subthalamic nucleus and external pallidum in basal ganglia circuitry. Brain Res Brain Res Rev 1995;20(1):128–54.

80. Shink E, Bevan MD, Bolam JP, et al. The subthalamic nucleus and the external pallidum: two tightly interconnected structures that control the output of the basal ganglia in the monkey. Neuroscience 1996;73(2):335–57.

81. Sato F, Parent M, Levesque M, et al. Axonal branching pattern of neurons of the subthalamic nucleus in primates. J Comp Neurol 2000;424(1):142–52.

82. Joel D, Weiner I. The connections of the primate subthalamic nucleus: indirect pathways and the open-interconnected scheme of basal ganglia-thalamocortical circuitry. Brain Res Brain Res Rev 1997;23(1–2):62–78.

83. Temel Y, Kessels A, Tan S, et al. Behavioural changes after bilateral subthalamic stimulation in advanced Parkinson disease: a systematic review. Parkinsonism Relat Disord 2006;12(5):265–72.

84. Smith Y, Hazrati LN, Parent A. Efferent projections of the subthalamic nucleus in the squirrel monkey as studied by the PHA-L anterograde tracing method. J Comp Neurol 1990;294(2):306–23.

85. Limousin P, Pollak P, Benazzouz A, et al. Bilateral subthalamic nucleus stimulation for severe Parkinson's disease. Mov Disord 1995;10(5):672–4.

86. Alvarez L, Macias R, Guridi J, et al. Dorsal subthalamotomy for Parkinson's disease. Mov Disord 2001;16(1):72–8.

87. Miller WC, Delong MR. Altered tonic activity of neurons in the globus pallidus and subthalamic nucleus in the primate MPTP model of Parkinsonism. In: Carpenter MB, Jayaraman A, editors. The Basal Ganglia, Vol 2, New York: Plenum Press; 1987. p. 415–27.

88. Bergman H, Wichmann T, DeLong MR. Reversal of experimental parkinsonism by lesions of the subthalamic nucleus. Science 1990;249(4975):1436–8.

89. Aziz TZ, Peggs D, Sambrook MA, et al. Lesion of the subthalamic nucleus for the alleviation of 1-methyl-4-phenyl-1,2,3,6-tetrahydropyridine (MPTP)-induced parkinsonism in the primate. Mov Disord 1991;6(4):288–92.

90. Bergman H, Wichmann T, Karmon B, et al. The primate subthalamic nucleus. II. Neuronal activity in the MPTP model of parkinsonism. J Neurophysiol 1994;72(2):507–20.

91. Wichmann T, Bergman H, DeLong MR. The primate subthalamic nucleus. I. Functional properties in intact animals. J Neurophysiol 1994;72(2):494–506.

92. Wichmann T, Bergman H, DeLong MR. The primate subthalamic nucleus. III. Changes in motor behavior and neuronal activity in the internal pallidum induced by subthalamic inactivation in the MPTP model of parkinsonism. J Neurophysiol 1994;72(2):521–30.

93. Limousin P, Pollak P, Benazzouz A, et al. Effect of parkinsonian signs and symptoms of bilateral subthalamic nucleus stimulation. Lancet 1995;345(8942):91–5.

94. Steele JC, Richardson JC, Olszewski J. Progressive supranuclear palsy. A heterogeneous degeneration involving the brain stem, basal ganglia and cerebellum with vertical gaze and pseudobulbar palsy, nuchal dystonia and dementia. Arch Neurol 1964;10:333–59.

95. Williams DR, Holton JL, Strand C, et al. Pathological tau burden and distribution distinguishes progressive supranuclear palsy-parkinsonism from Richardson's syndrome. Brain 2007;130(Pt 6):1566–76.

96. Gibb WR, Luthert PJ, Marsden CD. Corticobasal degeneration. Brain 1989;112(Pt 5):1171–92.

97. Geddes JF, Hughes AJ, Lees AJ, et al. Pathological overlap in cases of parkinsonism associated with neurofibrillary tangles. A study of recent cases of postencephalitic parkinsonism and comparison with progressive supranuclear palsy and Guamanian parkinsonism-dementia complex. Brain 1993; 116(Pt 1):281–302.

98. Schaltenbrand G, Wahren W. Atlas for Stereotaxy of the Human Brain. Stuttgart, New York: Thieme; 1977.

99. Zonenshayn M, Rezai AR, Mogilner AY, et al. Comparison of anatomic and neurophysiological methods for subthalamic nucleus targeting. Neurosurgery 2000;47(2):282–92 [discussion: 292–4].

100. Hamani C, Richter EO, Andrade-Souza Y, et al. Correspondence of microelectrode mapping with magnetic resonance imaging for subthalamic nucleus procedures. Surg Neurol 2005;63(3): 249–53 [discussion: 253].

101. Chen CC, Pogosyan A, Zrinzo LU, et al. Intraoperative recordings of local field potentials can help localize the subthalamic nucleus in Parkinson's disease surgery. Exp Neurol 2006;198(1): 214–21.

102. Lee C, Young B, Sanders MF. The role of the supramammillary commissure in MR localization of the subthalamic nucleus. Stereotact Funct Neurosurg 2006;84(5–6):193–204.

103. Counelis GJ, Simuni T, Forman MS, et al. Bilateral subthalamic nucleus deep brain stimulation for advanced PD: correlation of intraoperative MER and postoperative MRI with neuropathological findings. Mov Disord 2003;18(9):1062–5.

104. Hariz M, Blomstedt P, Limousin P. The myth of microelectrode recording in ensuring a precise location of the DBS electrode within the sensorimotor part of the subthalamic nucleus. Mov Disord 2004;19(7):863–4.

105. McClelland S 3rd, Vonsattel JP, Garcia RE, et al. Relationship of clinical efficacy to postmortem-determined anatomic subthalamic stimulation in Parkinson syndrome. Clin Neuropathol 2007; 26(6):267–75.

106. den Dunnen WF, Staal MJ. Anatomical alterations of the subthalamic nucleus in relation to age: a postmortem study. Mov Disord 2005;20(7):893–8.

107. Ashkan K, Blomstedt P, Zrinzo L, et al. Variability of the subthalamic nucleus: the case for direct MRI guided targeting. Br J Neurosurg 2007;21(2): 197–200.

108. Patel NK, Khan S, Gill SS. Comparison of atlas- and magnetic-resonance-imaging-based stereotactic targeting of the subthalamic nucleus in the surgical treatment of Parkinson's disease. Stereotact Funct Neurosurg 2008;86(3):153–61.

109. Davies KG, Daniluk S. Stereotactic targeting of the subthalamic nucleus: relevance of magnetic resonance-based evaluation of interindividual variation in diencephalic anatomy. Stereotact Funct Neurosurg 2008;86(5):330–1.

110. Richter EO, Hoque T, Halliday W, et al. Determining the position and size of the subthalamic nucleus based on magnetic resonance imaging results in patients with advanced Parkinson disease. J Neurosurg 2004;100(3):541–6.

111. Menuel C, Garnero L, Bardinet E, et al. Characterization and correction of distortions in stereotactic magnetic resonance imaging for bilateral subthalamic stimulation in Parkinson disease. J Neurosurg 2005;103(2):256–66.

112. Taoka T, Hirabayashi H, Nakagawa H, et al. "Sukeroku sign" and "dent internal-capsule sign"–identification guide for targeting the subthalamic nucleus for placement of deep brain stimulation electrodes. Neuroradiology 2009;51(1):11–6.

113. Andrade-Souza YM, Schwalb JM, Hamani C, et al. Comparison of three methods of targeting the subthalamic nucleus for chronic stimulation in Parkinson's disease. Neurosurgery 2005;56(Suppl 2): 360–8 [discussion: 360–68].

114. Rijkers K, Temel Y, Visser-Vandewalle V, et al. The microanatomical environment of the subthalamic nucleus. Technical note. J Neurosurg 2007; 107(1):198–201.

115. Toda H, Sawamoto N, Hanakawa T, et al. A novel composite targeting method using high-field magnetic resonance imaging for subthalamic nucleus deep brain stimulation. J Neurosurg 2009;111(4):737–45.

116. Yelnik J, Bardinet E, Dormont D, et al. A three-dimensional, histological and deformable atlas of the human basal ganglia. I. Atlas construction based on immunohistochemical and MRI data. Neuroimage 2007;34(2):618–38.

117. Bardinet E, Bhattacharjee M, Dormont D, et al. A three-dimensional histological atlas of the human basal ganglia. II. Atlas deformation strategy and evaluation in deep brain stimulation for Parkinson disease. J Neurosurg 2009;110(2):208–19.

118. Slavin KV, Thulborn KR, Wess C, et al. Direct visualization of the human subthalamic nucleus with 3T MR imaging. AJNR Am J Neuroradiol 2006;27(1):80–4.

119. Kitajima M, Korogi Y, Kakeda S, et al. Human subthalamic nucleus: evaluation with high-resolution MR imaging at 3.0 T. Neuroradiology 2008;50(8): 675–81.

120. Thomas DL, De Vita E, Roberts S, et al. High-resolution fast spin echo imaging of the human brain at 4.7 T: implementation and sequence characteristics. Magn Reson Med 2004;51(6):1254–64.

121. Bourekas EC, Christoforidis GA, Abduljalil AM, et al. High resolution MRI of the deep gray nuclei

at 8 Tesla. J Comput Assist Tomogr 1999;23(6):
867–74.

122. Volz S, Hattingen E, Preibisch C, et al. Reduction of
susceptibility-induced signal losses in multigradient-echo images: application to improved
visualization of the subthalamic nucleus. Neuroimage 2009;45(4):1135–43.

123. Elolf E, Bockermann V, Gringel T, et al. Improved visibility of the subthalamic nucleus on high-resolution
stereotactic MR imaging by added susceptibility
(T2*) contrast using multiple gradient echoes.
AJNR Am J Neuroradiol 2007;28(6):1093–4.

124. Vertinsky AT, Coenen VA, Lang DJ, et al. Localization of the subthalamic nucleus: optimization with
susceptibility-weighted phase MR imaging. AJNR
Am J Neuroradiol 2009;30(9):1717–24.

125. Manova ES, Habib CA, Boikov AS, et al. Characterizing the mesencephalon using susceptibility-
weighted imaging. AJNR Am J Neuroradiol 2009;
30(3):569–74.

126. Suhyadhom A, Haq IU, Foote KD, et al. A high resolution and high contrast MRI for differentiation of subcortical structures for DBS targeting: the fast gray matter
acquisition T1 inversion recovery (FGATIR). Neuroimage 2009;doi:10.1016/j.neuroimage.2009.04.018.

127. Price S, Paviour D, Scahill R, et al. Voxel-based
morphometry detects patterns of atrophy that
help differentiate progressive supranuclear palsy
and Parkinson's disease. Neuroimage 2004;23(2):
663–9.

128. Salamon N, Sicotte N, Alger J, et al. Analysis of the
brain-stem white-matter tracts with diffusion tensor
imaging. Neuroradiology 2005;47:895–902.

129. Wakana S, Jiang H, Nagae-Poetscher LM, et al.
Fiber tract-based atlas of human white matter
anatomy. Radiology 2004;230:77–87.

130. Nagae-Poetscher LM, Jiang H, Wakana S, et al.
High-resolution diffusion tensor imaging of the
brain stem at 3 T. AJNR Am J Neuroradiol 2004;
25:1325–30.

131. Stieltjes B, Kaufmann WE, van Zijl PC, et al. Diffusion tensor imaging and axonal tracking in the
human brainstem. Neuroimage 2001;14:723–35.

132. Nilsson C, Markenroth Bloch K, Brockstedt S, et al.
Tracking the neurodegeneration of parkinsonian
disorders–a pilot study. Neuroradiology 2007;49:
111–9.

133. Aravamuthan BR, Stein JF, Aziz TZ. The anatomy
and localization of the pedunculopontine nucleus
determined using probabilistic diffusion tractography. [corrected]. Br J Neurosurg 2008;22:
S25–32.

134. Muthusamy KA, Aravamuthan BR, Kringelbach ML,
et al. Connectivity of the human pedunculopontine
nucleus region and diffusion tensor imaging in
surgical targeting. J Neurosurg 2007;107:814–20.

135. Aravamuthan BR, Muthusamy KA, Stein JF, et al.
Topography of cortical and subcortical connections of the human pedunculopontine and subthalamic nuclei. Neuroimage 2007;37:694–705.

136. Johansen-Berg H, Behrens TE, Sillery E, et al.
Functional-anatomical validation and individual
variation of diffusion tractography-based segmentation of the human thalamus. Cereb Cortex 2005;
15:31–9.

137. Behrens TE, Johansen-Berg H, Woolrich MW, et al.
Non-invasive mapping of connections between
human thalamus and cortex using diffusion
imaging. Nat Neurosci 2003;6:750–7.

138. Zrinzo L, Zrinzo LV. Surgical anatomy of the pedunculopontine and peripeduncular nuclei. Br J Neurosurg 2008;22(Suppl 1):S19–24.

Brain Magnetic Resonance Imaging Techniques in the Diagnosis of Parkinsonian Syndromes

Klaus Seppi, MD*, Werner Poewe, MD

KEYWORDS

- Parkinson's disease • Atypical parkinsonism
- Magnetic resonance imaging (MRI)
- Diffusion weighted and diffusion tensor imaging (DW/DT)
- Magnetic resonance spectroscopy (MRS)
- Magnetization transfer imaging (MTI) • MR volumetry

Parkinson disease (PD) is the most common neurodegenerative cause of parkinsonism, followed by progressive supranuclear palsy (PSP) and multiple system atrophy (MSA). Despite the publication of consensus operational criteria[1–5] for the diagnosis of PD and the various atypical parkinsonian disorders (APD) such as PSP, MSA—especially the Parkinson variant of MSA (MSA-P)—and corticobasal degeneration (CBD), differentiation of these clinical entities may be challenging, particularly in the early stages of the disease, where overlapping clinical signs lead to a high rate of misclassification. Indeed, clinicopathologic series have revealed error rates for a clinical diagnosis of PD during life of up to 24% even in the hands of experienced neurologists.[5–10] On the other hand, diagnosis of PD and its distinction from APD and symptomatic parkinsonism are crucial for clinical evaluation, as these disorders differ in prognosis, treatment response, and molecular pathogenesis.[11–20]

This article focuses on static or structural magnetic resonance (MR) techniques such as conventional MR (cMR) imaging, including standard T2-, T1-weighted, and proton-density sequences, as well as different advanced MR imaging techniques, including methods to assess regional cerebral atrophy quantitatively such as magnetic resonance volumetry (MRV), diffusion-weighted and diffusion tensor (DW/DT) imaging, and magnetization transfer (MT) imaging, to assist in the differential diagnosis of neurodegenerative parkinsonian disorders. Except for MR spectroscopy (MRS), functional MR imaging techniques including perfusion MR imaging (PW-MR imaging) and blood oxygenation level-dependent (BOLD) functional MR imaging, which are mainly experimental and only of limited usefulness for diagnostic aspects in a parkinsonian patient, are not covered here. For the review, the authors systematically searched PubMed from 1983 until May 2009 by using a highly sensitive though arduous search strategy[21] adding the terms "brain," "magnetic resonance imaging," "MRI", "magnetic*," "DWI," "DTI," "diffusion," "diffusion*," "tensor," "volumetry," "MRV," "VBM," "voxel based morphometry," "voxel*," "spectroscopy," "MRS," "imaging," "atrophy," "diagnosis," "diagnos*," combined with "PD," "APD," "MSA," "PSP," "CBD," "CBS," "Richardson

Financial disclosure: The investigators have nothing to disclose in relation to this article.
Department of Neurology, Innsbruck Medical University, Anichstrasse 35, A-6020 Innsbruck, Austria
* Corresponding author.
E-mail address: klaus.seppi@uki.at (K. Seppi).

Neuroimag Clin N Am 20 (2010) 29–55
doi:10.1016/j.nic.2009.08.016

neuroimaging.theclinics.com

disease," "Richardson*," "atypical parkin-sonism," "parkinsonism," "neurodegenerative," "Parkinson's disease," "parkinson*," "multiple system atrophy," "multiple system," "supranu-clear," "akinesia," "progressive supranuclear palsy," "corticobasal degeneration," "cortico-basal," "corticobasal syndrome," using free text or MESH terms, or both where appropriate. Only articles published in English were considered for the review.

BRAIN MAGNETIC RESONANCE IMAGING TECHNIQUES

Since the early 1980s, MR imaging has been established in the routine diagnostic workup of neurologic disorders. The publication of 2 MR imaging studies on neurodegenerative parkin-sonism in the same issue of the journal *Radiology* in 1986, dealing with Parkinson plus syndromes,[22,23] represents the starting point for an increasing interest in different MR imaging techniques for the differential diagnosis in neurodegenerative parkin-sonian disorders.

The principles of MR imaging are based on the ubiquitous presence of hydrogen in body tissues and the spin of the hydrogen atom proton, which induces a small magnetic field. In general, T2-weighted sequences are sensitive to changes in tissue properties, including tissue damage, due to changes of the transverse magnetization or T2 decay.[24] Therefore, neurodegenerative processes characterized by cell loss, increased age-related deposition of iron or other paramagnetic substances, and by astroglial reaction and microglial proliferation may lead to signal changes in affected brain areas, like the basal ganglia or infratentorial structures, in neurodegenerative parkinsonism.[25–28] Due to a lengthening of the T2 decay, gliosis increases signal intensity on T2-weighted imaging, consistent with findings in a postmortem case of MSA, where brain areas with the most pronounced microgliosis and astro-gliosis correlated with the areas of hyperintense signal changes on MR imaging during life.[29] Nonheme iron in ferritin and hemosiderin in the brain are visualized by MR imaging due to selective shortening of T2 but not T1 relaxation time, thus leading to signal loss and hypointensity on T2-weighted images with minimal or no intensity change on T1 images. The sensitivity for signal changes due to iron deposition in the brain can be increased by using T2*-weighted gradient echo sequences or susceptibility weighted contrasts, or by applying conventional spin echo instead of fast spin echo T2-weighted scans.[30–32] Signal changes on T2-weighted images in the basal

ganglia as well as in infratentorial structures have been reported for all APDs at 1.5 T, where they have been used as a differentiating criterion from PD. However, whereas hyperintense putaminal rims at T2-weighted images at 1.5 T are common in MSA-P and rare in PD or healthy controls, a hyperintense putaminal rim on T2-weighted images at 3.0 T seems to be a nonspecific, normal finding.[33] When discussing signal changes at T2-weighted images in parkinsonian disorders here, the authors refer to 1.5 T field strengths, which is still the most commonly used technique in clinical routine and for which the most data are available.

T1-weighted sequences are important for anatomic details and provide good gray matter/white matter contrast. By using an inversion pulse, the contrast of T1-weighted images can be improved as in a magnetization-prepared rapid acquisition with gradient echo (MP-RAGE) sequence of high-resolution 3-dimensional (3D) datasets.[34] Another attempt to improve gray versus white matter differentiation makes use of a ratio of images acquired by 2 distinct inversion recovery sequences, which depends only on T1, one designed to suppress white matter and the other to suppress gray matter.[35,36] The combina-tion of these pulse sequences for inversion recovery ratio imaging has been postulated to be sensitive to cell loss, and was used in an attempt to image structural changes within the substantia nigra.[35,36]

As an indirect measure of brain structures known to be atrophic in different parkinsonian disorders, different groups have applied simple quantitative measures of diameters, areas, and volumes of different structures on MR imaging for the differen-tial diagnosis of neurodegenerative parkinsonism. More recently, voxel-based morphometry (VBM) has aroused interest in detecting volume loss in neurodegenerative parkinsonism. VBM is based on coregistration of high-resolution 3D datasets as obtained by MP-RAGE sequences, which are normalized to a study-specific template for detec-tion of volume differences between 2 or more groups. Contrary to operator-dependent segmen-tation techniques including region of interest (ROI) selection, VBM permits an operator-independent and automated detection of significant differences in different tissue types of the whole brain, involving voxel-wise statistical analysis of preprocessed structural MR images.[37] Voxel-based relaxometry (VBR) is a technique based on voxel-by-voxel calculation of whole brain T2 relaxation rate (R2) maps derived from multi-echo T2-weighted images to assess signal abnormalities.[38,39] However, as VBM and VBR involves groupwise comparisons, at this time it is not appropriate for routine diagnostic workup of individual patients. Further-more, in performing a voxel-based study many methodological options are available and known for pitfalls, which are summarized in a recent review.[40]

DW/DT imaging visualizes the random movement of water molecules in the tissue by applying diffusion-sensitizing gradients to assess changes in diffusion magnitude and orientation of water molecules in tissue. Quantification of the diffusivity is achieved by applying diffusion-sensitizing gradients of different degrees in 3 orthogonal directions and calculating the apparent diffusion coefficient (ADC) for each direction. The ADC is very dependent on the direction of diffusion encoding. To overcome this limitation, one can perform 3 orthogonal measurements and average the results to obtain a better approximation of the diffusion coefficient. This method is equivalent to the derivation of the trace from the diffusion tensor (Trace(D)). Therefore, the Trace(D) is sometimes also called averaged ADC (ADCave) or mean diffusivity. The random translational motion (diffusion) of water molecules in tissue is restricted by the highly organized architecture of fiber tracts in the central nervous system. Neuronal loss and gliosis disrupt this architecture, resulting in an increase of diffusivity and ADC. The complex neuronal architecture with its organization in fiber bundles that are surrounded by dense myelin sheaths leads also to a distinct anisotropy of water diffusion, which is facilitated along the direction of fiber tracts and restricted perpendicular to the fibers. The degree of anisotropy can be quantified by applying diffusion-sensitizing gradients in at least 6 directions, which permits calculation of fractional anisotropy (FA). Decreased FA values represent tissue degeneration due to normal aging or due to pathologic reasons such as neurodegeneration. Both diffusivity and FA can be combined to form the so-called diffusion tensor, which indicates direction and extent of diffusivity with the help of a vector.[41–43]

MT imaging is based on the interactions between bound protons within structures as myelin or cell membranes and the mobile protons of free water.[44] In MT imaging, a new contrast, depending on the exchange rate between coupled and free water protons, is induced by application of radiofrequency pulses that selectively destroy the magnetization of bound protons whereas free protons are unaffected. This process leads in turn to a decrease of the free water signal as exchange between free and bound water protons increases. The difference between signal intensities with and without MT is measured by calculating the MT ratios (MTRs), which correlate with the density of macromolecules, which are clearly reduced in demyelinated lesions and neurodegeneration.[45] However, most studies using MTR do not account for T1 relaxation, which can modulate MT rates and thus lead to ambiguous results.[46]

In proton magnetic resonance spectroscopy (^{1}H-MRS), protons chemically bound to different molecules can be differentiated by characteristic imprints of spectral resonances, the so-called chemical shifts.[47] The main resonances in brain ^{1}H-MRS relate to N-acetylaspartate (NAA) as an indirect expression of the integrity and function of neurons, choline (Cho)-containing compounds as marker for cell membrane turnover indicating glial activity, creatine (Cr)-including phosphocreatine as a marker for energy metabolism, as well as lactate as an indicator for anaerobic glycolysis detected under pathologic conditions.[48,49]

DIAGNOSIS OF NEURODEGENERATIVE PARKINSONIAN SYNDROMES WITH DIFFERENT MAGNETIC RESONANCE IMAGING TECHNIQUES
Conventional MR Imaging

In PD, standard T2-weighted, T1-weighted, and proton-density sequences at 1.5 T do not show disease-specific changes. Because cMR imaging is usually normal in early PD, cMR imaging takes a major part in excluding underlying pathologies such as vascular lesions, multiple sclerosis, brain tumors, normal pressure hydrocephalus, bilateral striopallidodentate calcinosis, and other potential, but rare causes of symptomatic parkinsonism such us Wilson disease, manganese-induced parkinsonism, or different subtypes of neurodegeneration associated with brain iron accumulation.[50–56] Furthermore, visual assessment of MR imaging can point toward alternative diagnosis from PD, when abnormalities that are characteristic of one of the APDs are seen (see later discussion and figures). At 1.5 T, patients with advanced PD, and sometimes those with APD, may show distinct abnormalities of the substantia nigra (SN), including signal increase on T2-weighted MR images or smudging of the hypointensity in the SN toward the red nucleus.[22,57–60] By using inversion recovery ratio imaging, structural changes in the SN have been reported in patients with PD.[35,36,61,62] Although some investigators were able to discriminate completely between PD patients and controls by using inversion recovery ratio imaging,[35,36] there was considerable overlap between normal and PD values in some of the studies published.[61,62]

Several findings on conventional structural MR imaging have been described as diagnostic pointers for MSA-P. These pointers include atrophy

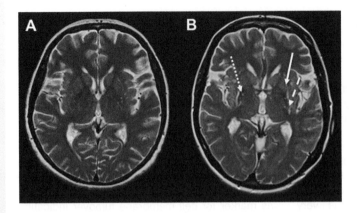

Fig. 1. Axial T2-weighted MR images at the striatal level in a patient with PD (*A*) and a patient with MSA-P (*B*). The image appears normal in the PD patient (*A*), whereas there is putaminal atrophy (*arrow*), putaminal hypointensity (*dotted arrow*), and a putaminal hyperintense rim (*dashed arrow*) in the patient with MSA-P (*B*).

and signal alterations (at 1.5 T) in the putamen (Fig. 1) and several infratentorial regions, such as the presence of a hyperintense putaminal rim with or without hypointensity in the dorsolateral part of the putamen, pontine atrophy, the "hot-cross bun" sign of the pons (Fig. 2), atrophy of the cerebellum, and hyperintensity in the middle cerebellar peduncle (MCP).[22,23,63–70] Whereas putaminal atrophy appears to discriminate MSA from PD, T2 putaminal hypointensity and a putaminal hyperintense rim may be observed also in PD.[68–72] In fact, on T2-weighted images at 3.0 T a hyperintense putaminal rim seems to be a nonspecific, normal finding.[33] Specificity of the aforementioned abnormalities to differentiate MSA-P from PD and healthy controls is considered high, whereas sensitivity, especially in the early disease stages, seems to

be insufficient.[60,70,73–75] Sensitivity of signal alterations, however, can be somewhat improved by modifying technical aspects such as spatial resolution by using thinner slices, or relaxation contrast by using conventional spin-echo (CSE) or T2*-weighted gradient echo sequences.[32,70,76,77]

Specific brain MR imaging findings associated with PSP include midbrain atrophy with enlargement of the third ventricle and tegmental atrophy, signal increase in the midbrain and in the inferior olives, atrophy of the superior cerebellar peduncle (SCP) as well as frontal and temporal lobe atrophy.[59,63,78–86] Indirect parameters of midbrain atrophy comprising reduced anteroposterior (AP) midbrain diameter, dilated third ventricle, and abnormal superior profile of the midbrain (flat or concave versus convex aspect in healthy people) may assist in the differential diagnosis of PSP.[60,87,88] Another indirect sign of midbrain atrophy in patients with PSP is the "penguin silhouette" or "hummingbird" sign (Fig. 3),[79,89,90] where the shape of the midbrain tegmentum (the bird's head) and pons (the bird's body) on midsagittal MR images resemble a lateral view of a standing king penguin or hummingbird.

Visual assessment of atrophy of the SCP has been shown to distinguish PSP patients from controls and patients with other parkinsonian disorders including MSA and PD, with a sensitivity of 74% and a specificity of 94%.[80] Moreover, some of the PSP patients may have increased signal changes in the SCP on fluid-attenuated inversion recovery (FLAIR) images, which seem to be absent in PD and MSA.[91]

In patients with CBD, only few studies have investigated the role of cMR imaging, showing cortical (especially frontoparietal) atrophy, which tends to be asymmetric, putaminal hypointensity as well as hyperintense signal changes in the motor cortex or

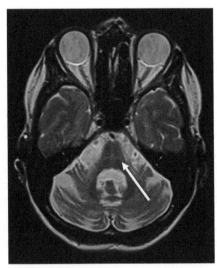

Fig. 2. Axial T2-weighted MR image in a patient with MSA-P, demonstrating the "hot-cross bun" sign (*arrow*) in the basis pontis.

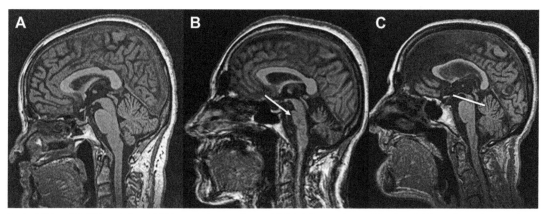

Fig. 3. Midsagittal T1-weighted MR images in a patient with PD (*A*), a patient with MSA-P (*B*), and a patient with PSP (*C*). (*A*) There is no pontine or midbrain atrophy in the patient with PD. (*B*) Pontine atrophy (*arrow*) without midbrain atrophy in the MSA-P patient. (*C*) Midbrain atrophy without pontine atrophy (divided by the *white line*) in the PSP patient, forming the silhouette of the "penguin" or "hummingbird" sign, with the shapes of midbrain tegmentum (bird's head; above the *white line*) and pons (bird's body; below the *white line*) looking like the lateral view of a standing penguin (especially the king penguin) or hummingbird, with a small head and big body.

subcortical white matter on T2-weighted images.[60,83,85,92,93] However, none of these cMR imaging abnormalities seems to be of diagnostic relevance for CBD.[83,93] Indeed, a review of 40 autopsy cases presenting with a corticobasal syndrome in life and with different pathologies at postmortem confirms that MR imaging findings are similar regardless of the differing underlying pathology.[93]

Overall, although specificity of cMR imaging for discriminating the different APDs from PD or healthy controls has been shown to be high, specificity of cMR imaging between the different APDs is inefficient.[33,60,63,68,70,73–75,83]

MR Planimetry and ROI-based MR Volumetry

As an indirect measure of brain structures known to be atrophic in different parkinsonian disorders, groups have applied simple quantitative measures of diameters and areas on MR imaging for the differential diagnosis of neurodegenerative parkinsonism. In terms of infratentorial atrophy, differentiation of PSP and MSA from each other and from PD have been based on studies showing that patients with PSP have relatively greater midbrain atrophy and greater SCP atrophy whereas, conversely, patients with MSA have relatively greater pontine and MCP atrophy.[79,80,87,88,94–96] A reduced AP midbrain diameter of less than 14 mm has been proposed to optimally separate PSP from other types of neurodegenerative parkinsonism and healthy controls,[88] whereas there were overlapping individual values in more recent studies.[87,95,96] The average MCP width was shown to be significantly smaller in patients with MSA than in those with PD or control subjects without any

overlap between MSA patients and PD patients or healthy subjects, using a cutoff value of 8 mm.[94] The separation of MSA from PSP patients, however, was inaccurate.[94,95] Consistent with the well-known atrophy of the pons in MSA, the area of the pons measured on midsagittal T1-weighted MR images has been shown to be smaller in MSA-P patients compared with patients with PD and PSP as well as healthy controls, albeit with some overlap at the individual level.[79,95] On the other hand, midbrain areas measured on midsagittal T1-weighted MR images are smaller in PSP patients compared with healthy controls and patients with PD and MSA-P.[79,95] Calculation of the ratio between pontine and midbrain areas has been demonstrated to discriminate completely between PSP patients and patients with PD, MSA-P, or healthy controls,[79] whereas there were overlapping individual values in another study.[95] For this reason, Quattrone and colleagues[95] proposed an index termed the MR parkinsonism index (MRPI), which was calculated by multiplying the ratio of pontine-to-midbrain area (P/M) by the ratio of the MCP-to-SCP width (MCP/SCP). The MRPI was significantly larger in patients with PSP than in healthy controls and patients with both PD and MSA-P, and completely separated PSP patients from the other groups,[95] such that further confirmatory studies seem warranted.

Volume loss of different supratentorial and infratentorial brain structures, measured by MRV with semi-automatic segmentation techniques on a ROI approach, has been reported in patients with MSA, PSP, and CBD.[63,81,97–100] On the other hand, most of the ROI-based MRV studies were not able to detect any volume differences in the basal ganglia, whole brain, infratentorial brain structures, or different brain lobes between PD patients and controls.[63,81,97,98,100,101] With advancing disease, however, hippocampal atrophy has been reported in patients with PD compared with healthy controls at a group level.[101-103]

Patients with MSA showed significant reductions in mean striatal, brainstem, and cerebellar volumes,[81,98,100] and patients with PSP showed significant reductions in whole brain, striatal, brainstem (especially midbrain), and frontal volumes.[81,97,99,100] Only one study used the volumetric approach in CBD, and found atrophy of the parietal cortex and corpus callosum.[99] The strength of this latter study is the use of post-mortem confirmed cases of PSP and CBD, and controls to construct a mathematical model derived from a discriminant analysis. The volumes of midbrain, parietal white matter, temporal gray matter, brainstem, frontal white matter, and pons were identified to separate best between groups predicting the diagnosis correctly in 95% of controls, as well as in 76% of all PSP and 83% of all CBD patients.

Voxel-based Morphometry and Relaxometry

More recently, VBM has aroused interest in detecting volume loss in neurodegenerative parkinsonism. Whereas most of the ROI-based MRV studies were not able to detect any volume differences between PD patients and controls,[97,98,100] various VBM studies revealed gray matter loss of frontal cortical areas, including motor areas, especially in advanced PD.[104-106]

In patients with MSA, VBM[38,39,107-109] confirmed previous ROI-based volumetric studies showing basal ganglia and infratentorial volume loss in MSA-P patients. Furthermore, these data also revealed volume loss in several cortical regions in patients with MSA-P and MSA-C. VBM has also been used to investigate the progression of cortical and subcortical atrophy patterns in MSA-P compared with PD,[110] and revealed early degeneration of the basal ganglia followed by later onset cortical atrophy.

Most recently, VBR was used to study brain morphology of MSA-C versus MSA-P and healthy volunteers.[38,39] In accordance to the VBM analysis in MSA-C that showed reductions of gray and white matter in the cerebellum and brainstem, VBR analysis revealed reduction of relaxation rate R2 in the same regions, reflecting infratentorial brain atrophy.[39] In addition, R2 was increased in the putamen, a region in which VBM did not show abnormalities, thus suggesting that the

combination of VBR and VBM may provide convergent and complementary information about the brain morphology of MSA-C.[39] Using VBM and VBR, direct comparison of MSA-C and MSA-P showed differences only in infratentorial brain regions where structural abnormalities were more pronounced in MSA-C than in MSA-P. In MSA-C, there was a stronger volume reduction of gray matter in the basal parts of the cerebellum and of white matter in the brainstem, as well as a stronger reduction of the relaxation rate R2 in the cerebellum and brainstem.[38]

By applying VBM, gray matter loss in PSP patients has been found in frontotemporal cortical areas such as the prefrontal cortex, the insular region comprising the frontal opercula, the supplementary motor areas, and the left mediotemporal area, whereas white matter loss has been additionally reported in the midbrain including cerebral peduncles and central midbrain.[111] A further study compared patients with PSP not only to controls but also to PD patients, and described a similar pattern of white matter volume loss in the midbrain comprising subthalamic region, cerebral peduncles, and midbrain tegmentum.[112] Of note, this latter study tested the clinical utility of the VBM results as a guide for the differential diagnosis of PSP from PD and controls by allocating the subject to either PSP or "non-PSP" based on the presence or absence of the midbrain tissue loss on T1-weighted images as detected by the VBM analysis, and achieved a sensitivity of 83% and a specificity of 79%.[112] A more recent study used VBM to compare neuroanatomical differences between clinically diagnosed PSP and CBD patients.[113] Midbrain structures were more atrophied in PSP than in CBD, whereas dorsal frontal and parietal cortices were more atrophied in CBD than in PSP.[113]

Diffusion-Weighted and Diffusion Tensor Imaging

Whereas earlier studies focusing on measures of diffusivity, but not FA, mainly in the midbrain and SN[43,70,114-118] did not find any differences between PD patients and healthy controls, several newer studies detected a decrease in FA in the SN in patients with PD compared with healthy controls.[119-121] This observation is in line with the well-known neurodegeneration of the SN in PD, although the exact mechanism of the reported FA changes is not known. Whereas FA measures could not identify PD patients on an individual basis consistently in 2 older studies using DT imaging at 1.5 T,[119,120] a recent study including only patients with newly diagnosed PD used high-resolution DT imaging at 3 T[121] to evaluate rostral, middle, and caudal ROIs within the SN on a single slice of the midbrain and this study found that PD patients could be completely separated from the control group based on reduced FA values in the caudal ROI of the SN, such that further confirmatory studies seem warranted.

Other groups drew attention by performing whole brain DT imaging analyses in patients with PD.[122,123] The finding of an increase of the 25th percentile of the whole brain FA histograms in patients with de novo PD compared with age-matched controls in the absence of total brain, gray matter, and white matter volume changes between the 2 groups was interpreted as subtle whole brain gray matter loss in patients with PD, even in the early clinical stages.[123] By using statistical parametric mapping analysis of DT imaging, changes in FA were found in the frontal lobes, including the supplementary motor area, the pre-supplementary motor area, and the cingulum in nondemented PD patients relative to controls, whereas VBM analysis in the same patients revealed no volume loss.[122] These results confirm that the neurodegenerative process extends beyond the basal ganglia in PD.[122,123]

By applying voxel-wise analysis on Trace(D) maps, MR structural changes of the olfactory tract were found in patients with PD,[124] a particularly intriguing finding given that hyposmia is present some 90% of patients with PD.

Over the past decade, there has been growing interest also in the use of DW/DT imaging for the differential diagnosis of APDs from PD. The most relevant studies are summarized in Table 1. Several studies performed on a ROI basis have shown that DW imaging permits discrimination between MSA-P in early disease stages and PD as well as healthy subjects, based on putaminal diffusivity measure values.[43,70,117,125–129] Whereas increased putaminal ADC and Trace(D) values (Fig. 4) overlapped in MSA-P and PSP patients,[117,130] abnormal diffusivity measures in the MCP[114,115,127,128,131] and SCP[114,116,130] have been reported for MSA and PSP, respectively, with some studies reporting a good differentiation of PSP and MSA from each other[115,130] or from controls, PD, or even corticobasal syndrome (CBS).[116,128,130]

Although most reports have found clearly increased putaminal diffusivity measures in MSA-P at 1.5 T,[43,70,125,127–129] there was one study which did not confirm this.[115] Methodological reasons (ie, segmentation error as demonstrated by a published figure where the delineated ROI of the putamen clearly contains parts of the globus pallidus and the thalamus is larger than that displayed; inadequate DW-MR protocol with a slice thickness of 7 mm compared with 2–5 mm used in other studies) and demographic (longer disease duration of the PD group) might explain this discrepancy.[117,127,128] The same study[115] also failed to detect diffusivity changes in the SCP of PSP patients, again in contrast with previous reports showing significantly increased diffusivity measures in the SCP in PSP patients[114,116,130] at 1.5 T. Although abnormal diffusivity in the MCP has been reported to have a high diagnostic accuracy for MSA-P in some articles,[115,128] this could not be confirmed by others.[114,127]

Of particular relevance to the use of MR imaging measures as biomarkers for disease progression, several studies have found a correlation of putaminal diffusivity measures with disease severity.[43,70,71,127]

Using 3.0 T in patients with MSA, PD, and controls, all patients that had both significantly low FA and high diffusivity values in the 3 areas studied (pons, putamen, and cerebellum) were MSA-P cases, and those that had both normal FA and Trace(D) values in the pons were all PD cases.[125] More recently, DW imaging has also been studied in patients with CBS, as summarized in Table 1.[116,132]

Magnetization Transfer Imaging

Abnormalities of the basal ganglia and SN by using MT imaging have been reported in patients with PD, MSA, and PSP.[133–135] It has been suggested that in patients with PD, MTR in the pars compacta of the SN is decreased at a group level, with overlapping individual values.[133–135] One study investigated the potential of MT imaging in the differential diagnosis of neurodegenerative parkinsonism, including 37 patients with different parkinsonian syndromes and 20 age-matched controls.[134] The main finding in this study was a change in the MTRs in the globus pallidus, putamen, caudate nucleus, SN, and white matter in PD, MSA, and PSP patients, matching the pathologic features of the underlying disorder. MTRs were significantly reduced in the putamen in MSA patients compared with PD patients and healthy controls, as well as in the SN in patients with PSP, MSA, and PD. By application of stepwise discriminant analysis, there was a good discrimination of PD patients and controls from the MSA and PSP patients, with only 1 out of 12 MSA patients wrongly classified into the control group. On the other hand, separation between PD patients and controls as well as between MSA and PSP patients was insufficient.[134]

Proton Magnetic Resonance Spectroscopy

Studies using ^{1}H-MRS have shown reduced NAA/Cr and NAA/Cho ratios in the lentiform nucleus or

Table 1
DW/DT imaging in atypical parkinsonism: summary of the available studies

Study, Year	Cohort Size/Methods	Results	Diagnostic Predictor	Sensitivity (%)	Specificity (%)
Schocke et al, 2002[70]	– MSA-P 10/PD 11/HC 7 – Assessment of ADC values (measured in the slice direction only) on a ROI basis in several ROIs (pons, SN, GP, CN, PUT, thalamus, GM, WM)	• Significant increased putaminal ADC values in MSA-P compared with PD and HC • No significant group differences of ADC values in the other ROIs • Significant correlation between UPDRS-III and putaminal ADC values	ADCs in the basal ganglia, pons, white matter; sensitivity and specificity values given for putaminal ADCs (best discriminator)		
			Putaminal ADCs > 0.760 × 10³ mm²/s	100 (MSA-P)	100 (vs PD and HC)
Seppi et al, 2003[117]	– MSA-P 12/PD 13/PSP 10 including all PD and MSA-P patients studied by Schocke et al, 2002[70] – Assessment of ADC values (measured in the slice direction only) on a ROI basis in several ROIs (pons, SN, GP, CN, PUT, thalamus, GM, WM)	• Significant increased ADCs in PUT, GP and CN in PSP compared with PD • No differences of ADC values of the different ROIs between PSP and MSA-P			
			Putaminal ADCs > 0.760 × 10³ mm²/s	100 (MSA-P)/90 (PSP)	100 (vs PD)

| Kanazawa et al, 2004[131] | – MSA-C 12/HC 11
– Assessment of ADC values (measured in the slice direction only) on a ROI basis in several ROIs (MCP, pons, CN, PUT, thalamus, cerebellar and parietal WM) | • Significant increased ADC values in the MCP, pons, putamen, and cerebellar WM in patients with MSA-C compared with HC
• Significant correlation of disease duration with ADC values in the MCP, pons, and cerebellar WM | | | |
| Seppi et al, 2004[118] | – MSA-P 15/PD 17/HC 10 including all PD and MSA-P patients as well as 2 of the HC studied by Schocke et al, 2002[70]
– Assessment of striatal ADCs and S/FC ratio using IBZM | • Significant lower S/FC ratios and higher striatal ADC values in MSA-P compared with both PD and HC
• No significant differences in S/FC ratios and striatal ADC values between PD and HC
• Higher overall predictive accuracy of striatal ADCs (97%) compared with S/FC ratio using IBZM (75%) | Striatal ADCs | Striatal ADCs > 0.795 $\times 10^3$ mm^2/s | 93 (MSA-P)   100 (vs PD and HC) |

(continued on next page)

Table 1
(continued)

Study, Year	Cohort Size/Methods	Results	Diagnostic Predictor	Sensitivity (%)	Specificity (%)
Schocke et al, 2004[43]	– MSA-P 11/PD 17/HC 10 – Assessment of ADC values (measured in the 3 orthogonal direction) and of the averaged ADC (Trace(D)) on a ROI basis in several ROIs (pons, SN, GP, CN, PUT, thalamus, GM, WM)	• Significant higher putaminal and pallidal ADC values in MSA-P compared with both PD patients and healthy volunteers • Complete discrimination between MSA-P vs PD and HC with putaminal Trace(D) values • Significant correlation between UPDRS-III and putaminal diffusivity	Putaminal diffusivity values		
			Putaminal Trace(D) > 0.80 × 10^3 mm²/s	100 (MSA-P)	100 (vs PD and HC)
Shiga et al, 2005[150]	– MSA 11/HC 10 – Assessment of FA-values in ICP, MCP, SCP, basis pontis, internal capsule, CC	• Significant decreased FA values in MCP, basis pontis, and internal capsule • Significant negative correlation of MCP FA values with ataxia scores			

Study	Methods	Findings	Measure	Sensitivity	Specificity
Seppi et al, 2006[129]	– MSA-P 15/PD 20/HC 11 including all patients studied by Schocke et al, 2004[43] – Assessment of ADC values in the entire, anterior, and posterior putamen	• Significant increased ADC values in the entire, anterior, and posterior putamen in MSA-P compared with PD and HC • Significant higher ADC values in the posterior putamen compared with the anterior putamen in MSA-P • No significant differences between ADC values in posterior and anterior putamen in PD and HC	Putaminal ADC values of the whole, anterior, and posterior putamen		
			Putaminal ADC > 0.80 $\times 10^3$ mm²/s	93 (MSA-P)	100 (vs PD and HC)
			Posterior putaminal ADC > 0.80 $\times 10^3$ mm²/s	100 (MSA-P)	100 (vs PD and HC)
Nicoletti et al, 2006[128]	– MSA-P 16/PD 16/PSP 16/HC 15 – Assessment of ADC values on a ROI basis in several ROIs (MCP, pons, GP, CN, PUT, thalamus, GM, WM)	• Significant increased putaminal ADC values in MSA-P compared with PD and HC • Significant increased MCP ADC values in MSA-P not only compared with PD and HC but also compared with PSP	ADC values in the basal ganglia, pons, white matter; sensitivity and specificity values given for putaminal and MCP diffusivity (best discriminators)		
			MCP ADC > 0.875 $\times 10^3$ mm²/s	100 (MSA-P)	100 (vs all groups)
			Putaminal ADC > 0.953 $\times 10^3$ mm²/s	100 (MSA-P)	100 (vs PD and HC) 81 (vs PSP)
			Putaminal ADC > 0.93 $\times 10^3$ mm²/s (estimated from Fig. 2 of the article)	75 (PSP)	97 (vs PD and HC) 100 (vs PD) 94 (vs HC)

(continued on next page)

Table 1
(continued)

Study, Year	Cohort Size/Methods	Results	Diagnostic Predictor	Sensitivity (%)	Specificity (%)
Blain et al, 2006[114]	– MSA-P 10/MSA-C 7/PD 12/ PSP 17/HC 12 – Assessment of ADC and FA values on a ROI basis in several ROIs (MCP, pons, decussation of SCP)	• Significant increased ADC and decreased FA values in MCP in MSA compared with PSP/PD/HC • Significant increased pontine ADC values in MSA compared with PSP/PD/HC • Significant increased SCP ADC values in PSP compared with MSA/PD/HC and significant decreased SCP FA values in PSP compared with PD • Significant correlation between ataxia scores and ADC values in MCP and pons in MSA			

| Padovani et al, 2006[151] | – PSP 14/HC 14
– VBM and whole brain voxel-wise analysis of FA | • VBM: Significant clusters of reduced GM in premotor cortex, frontal operculum, anterior insula, hippocampus, and parahippocampal gyrus, bilaterally; and with regard to subcortical brain regions, significant tissue loss in the pulvinar, dorsomedial, and anterior nuclei of the thalamus, and superior and inferior colliculus, bilaterally
• Voxel-wise FA analysis: reduced FA in superior longitudinal fasciculus, anterior part of CC, arcuate fasciculus, posterior thalamic radiations, and internal capsule |
| Nilsson et al, 2007[152] | – MSA-P 4/PD 2/PSP 3/HC 2
– Tractography and assessment of ADC and FA values in SCP and MCP without statistical analysis | • Degeneration of the MCP and pontine crossing tracts, with decreased FA and increased ADC in advanced MSA
• Selective degeneration of the SCP in PSP |

(continued on next page)

Table 1
(continued)

Study, Year	Cohort Size/Methods	Results	Diagnostic Predictor	Sensitivity (%)	Specificity (%)
Köllensperger et al, 2007[126]	– MSA-P 9/PD 9/HC 16 – Assessment of putaminal ADC values, H/M ratio and tilt table testing	• Significant increased putaminal ADC values in MSA-P compared with PD and HC • Significant lower H/M ratios in PD compared with HC with considerable overlap between MSA-P and PD • No significant differences of blood pressure response to passive tilt between PD and MSA-P • DW imaging superior to both tilt table testing and MIBG scintigraphy in the differential diagnosis of PD vs MSA-P	Putaminal ADC values		
Paviour et al, 2007[115]	– MSA-P 11/PD 12/PSP 20/HC 7 – Assessment of ADC values on a ROI basis in several ROIs (MCP, caudal and rostral pons, midbrain, decussation of SCP, thalamus, GP, CN, PUT, CC, frontal and parietal WM, centrum semiovale)	• Significant higher ADC values in the MCP and rostral pons in MSA-P compared with PSP and PD • Significant correlation between ADC values in rostral pons and H&Y in MSA-P • Significant correlation between GP ADC values and H&Y and UPDRS-II and -III in PSP	Putaminal ADC > 0.79 × 10³ mm²/s ADC values in the basal ganglia, pons, MCP, SCP, thalamus; sensitivity and specificity values given for MCP diffusivity (in the article)	100 (MSA-P)	100 (vs all groups)

		MCP ADC > 0.733 $\times 10^3$ mm²/s	91 (MSA-P)	82 (vs all groups)/ 84 (vs PSP)
Ito et al, 2007[125]	– MSA 20 (MSA-P 10)/PD 21/ HC 20 – Assessment of ADC and FA values on a ROI basis in the pons, cerebellum and putamen at 3.0 T	• Significant higher ADC and significant lower FA values in the pons, cerebellum, and putamen in MSA compared with PD/HC • No difference in the ADC and FA values of the different regions between MSA-P and MSA-C • All patients that had both significant low FA and high ADC values in each of the 3 regions were MSA-P cases, and those that had both normal FA and ADC values in the pons were all PD cases	FA and ADC in the pons, cerebellum, and putamen at 3.0 T; sensitivity and specificity values given for MSA-P10 vs PD		
			ADC pons > 0.98 $\times 10^3$ mm²/s	70	70
			ADC cerebellum > 0.96 $\times 10^3$ mm²/s	60	88
			ADC putamen > 0.83 $\times 10^3$ mm²/s	70	64
			FA pons < 0.38	70	100
			FA cerebellum < 0.30	70	64
			FA putamen < 0.35	70	88
			both low FA and high ADC values in any of the 3 areas	90	100

(continued on next page)

Table 1
(*continued*)

Study, Year	Cohort Size/Methods	Results	Diagnostic Predictor	Sensitivity (%)	Specificity (%)
Nicoletti et al, 2008[130]	− MSA-P 15/PD 16/PSP 15 including all patients studied by Nicoletti et al, 2006[128] − Assessment of ADC values in the SCP	• Significant higher SCP ADC values in PSP compared with MSA-P, PD, and HC	SCP ADC values		
			SCP ADC > 0.943 × 10³ mm²/s	100 (PSP)	93 (vs PD and MSA-P)/100 (vs HC) 100 (vs PD) 87 (vs MSA-P)
Rizzo et al, 2008[116]	− PSP 10/CBS 7/PD 13/HC 9 − Assessment of ADC values on a ROI basis in several ROIs (midbrain, CC, SCP, GP, CN, PUT, thalamus, posterior limb of internal capsule, frontal and parietal WM). Generation of histograms of ADCs (with determination of medians) for all voxels in left and right cerebral hemispheres and in left and right deep gray matter regions separately to calculate the ratio of the smaller to the larger median value (symmetry ratio) for left and right hemispheres and for left and right deep gray matter regions (1 = perfect symmetry)	• Significant higher putaminal ADC values in PSP and CBS compared with PD and HC • Significant higher SCP ADC values in PSP compared with CBS, PD, and HC • Significant increased higher valued hemispheric median ADC values of the cerebral hemispheric histograms in CBS compared with PSP, PD, and HC • Complete discrimination between CBS and the other groups based on the hemispheric symmetry ratio	ADC values of all ROIs, medians of left and right cerebral hemispheres and of left and right deep gray matter regions, and symmetry ratios for both hemispheres and deep gray matter regions; sensitivity and specificity values given for best discriminators		
			Putaminal ADC > 0.745 × 10³ mm²/s	86 (CBS)	91 (vs HC and PD) 92 (vs PD)

	Putaminal ADC > 0.735 × 10³ mm²/s	80 (PSP)	82 (vs HC and PD) / 77 (vs PD)
	SCP ADC > 0.815 × 10³ mm²/s	90 (PSP)	75 (vs all groups) / 91 (vs HC and PD) / 85 (vs PD)
	Median ADC in the higher valued hemisphere > 0.925 × 10³ mm²/s	86 (CBS)	81 (vs all groups) / 77 (vs HC and PD) / 85 (vs PD) / 90 (vs PSP)
	Median ADC in the higher valued hemisphere > 0.895 × 10³ mm²/s	100 (CBS)	72 (vs all groups) / 64 (vs HC and PD) / 62 (vs PD) / 90 (vs PSP)
	Hemispheric symmetry ratio > 0.981	100 (CBS)	100 (CBS)
Boelmans et al, 2008[132]	– CBS 10/HC 10 – Application of fiber tractography and DT imaging to analyze the axonal integrity of white matter projections, namely corticospinal and transcallosal motor projections		• Reduced fiber projections in the corticospinal tract on the first affected side as well as in the CC, particularly in the posterior trunk, in CBS compared with HC with significantly increased ADC and reduced FA values in these regions in CBS compared with HC

(continued on next page)

Table 1
(continued)

Study, Year	Cohort Size/Methods	Results	Diagnostic Predictor	Sensitivity (%)	Specificity (%)
Pellecchia et al, 2009[127]	– MSA-P 9/MSA-C 12/HC 11 – Assessment of ADC values on a ROI basis in several ROIs (MCP, pons, anterior and posterior PUT, entire PUT, CN, cerebellar WM)	• Significant increased ADC values in entire and anterior PUT in MSA-P compared with MSA-C/HC • Significant increased ADC values in posterior PUT in MSA-P compared with HC • Significant increased ADC values in MCP and cerebellar WM in MSA-C compared with MSA-P/HC • Significant increased pontine ADC values in MSA-C compared with HC • Significant higher ADC values in the posterior compared with the anterior putamen in MSA-P and MSA-C, but not in PD and HC • Significant correlation of disease duration with cerebellar ADC values in MSA-C and pontine ADC values in MSA-P • Significant correlation of UMSARS and UPDRS with ADC values in posterior and entire putamen			

| Tir et al, 2009[153] | – MSA-P 14/PD 19/HC 14
– VBM and whole brain voxel-wise analysis of FA | • VBM: significant lower density of GM in MSA-P in a motor-related circuit, especially in the left primary motor cortex, relative to PD, and in the left supplementary motor area, relative to HC
• Voxel-wise FA analysis: significant reduced FA in the left primary motor cortex and the right cerebellum
• No clinicoradiological correlation with FA values |

Abbreviations: CBS, corticobasal syndrome; HC, healthy controls; MSA, multiple system atrophy; MSA-P, Parkinson variant of MSA; PD, Parkinson disease; PSP, progressive supranuclear palsy.

ADC, apparent diffusion coefficient—in the studies by Schocke et al, 2002,[70] Seppi et al, 2003,[117] Seppi et al, 2004,[118] and Kanazawa et al, 2004[131] measured in z-slice direction only, in the other studies ADCs were averaged over 3 orthogonal measurements, thus representing the trace of the diffusion tensor (Trace (D)); FA, fractional anisotropy; H/M ratio, activity ratio of heart to mediastinum uptake for cardiac MIBG (meta-iodobenzylguanidine) scintigraphy; IBZM, [^{123}I]iodobenzamide; S/FC ratio, activity ratios of striatal to frontal cortex uptake.

CC, corpus callosum; CN, caudate nucleus; GM, gray matter; GP, globus pallidus; ICP, inferior cerebellar peduncle; MCP, middle cerebellar peduncle; PUT, putamen; SCP, superior cerebellar peduncle; SN, substantia nigra; WM, white matter.

H&Y, Hoehn and Yahr stage; UMSARS, Unified MSA Rating Scale; UPDRS, Unified PD Rating Scale.

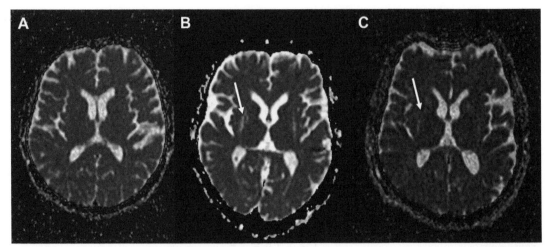

Fig. 4. Axial Trace(D) maps at the level of mid-striatum in a patient with PD (*A*), a patient with MSA-P (*B*), and a patient with PSP (*C*). Note the diffuse hyperintensity, corresponding to increased Trace(D) values, in the putamen (*arrows*) in the patients with MSA-P (*B*) and PSP (*C*).

striatum, not only in APD but also in PD,[48,136–141] disproving previously published results that suggested that ^{1}H-MRS of striatal structures might differentiate APDs from PD by virtue of reduced NAA/Cr ratios in MSA but not PD.[138,139] Technical factors, including the application of different echo and relaxation times, voxel sizes, and pulse sequences, mostly may account for some of the contradictory results.[48,137]

The development of ^{1}H-MRS at higher magnetic field strengths may lead ^{1}H-MRS to a more important role as imaging tool in the differential

Table 2
Brain MR features in neurodegenerative parkinsonism

Brain MR Feature	PD	MSA-P	PSP	Refs.
cMR imaging				
Normal (in the age range)	++	−	−	32,64,67,68,70,72,78a
Putaminal atrophy	−	++	++	64,68,70,72,83a
Putaminal hyperintense rim at 1.5 T	+	++	+	64,67–70,72,75,83a
Putaminal hypointensity at 1.5 T	−	++	−	32,64,67,68,70,72,83a
Pontine and cerebellar vermian atrophy	−	++	+	64,72,75,83a
Signal changes in the pons or MCP including "hot-cross bun" sign at 1.5 T	−	++	−	64,66,75,83a
Midbrain atrophy including indirect signs of midbrain atrophy	−	−	++	59,72,78,80,83,87a
MR planimetry				
Reduced AP midbrain diameter	−	+	++	78,83,87,88
Reduced ratio between midbrain and pontine areas	−	−	+++	79,95,96
DW/DT imaging				
Increased putaminal diffusivity at 1.5 T	−	+++	++	43,70,116–118,126–129
Increased SCP diffusivity at 1.5 T	−	−	+++	114,116,128

−, <20%; +, 20%–50%; ++, 50%–70%; +++, 70%–90%; ++++, >90%. Only MR imaging findings that have been confirmed by at least 2 concordant studies are listed.

Abbreviations: AP, anterior-posterior; MCP, middle cerebellar peduncle; MSA-P, Parkinson variant of multiple system atrophy; PD, Parkinson disease (early disease stages); PSP, progressive supranuclear palsy (referred to as Richardson disease); SCP, superior cerebellar peduncle.

[a] Not all available studies cited.

diagnosis of parkinsonian disorders. ^{1}H-MRS at higher magnetic field strengths increases sensitivity and dispersion of the chemical shift, even though greater magnetic susceptibility may diminish this benefit. A recent study applied multiple regional single-voxel ^{1}H-MRS including putamen, pontine base, and cerebral white matter at 3.0 T in 24 patients with MSA compared with 11 PD patients and 18 controls.[142] In both MSA-C and MSA-P significant NAA/Cr reductions were shown in the pontine base, whereas reduced putaminal NAA/Cr was found in the patients with MSA-P. There was a significant NAA/Cr reduction in the pontine base as well as in the putamen in patients with MSA-P compared with both controls and PD, which suggests that the combined assessment of NAA/Cr in the pontine base and putamen may help to distinguish MSA-P from PD.[142]

LIMITATIONS

The characteristic imaging abnormalities described in the different types of neurodegenerative parkinsonism rely on studies in patients whose clinical diagnosis is based on clinical diagnostic criteria as gold standard without pathologic confirmation, such that misdiagnosis in some of the clinically diagnosed patients cannot be excluded[5–10] and generalization of the findings might be limited. As diagnostic certainty increases with disease progression,[143–145] most of the studies have included patients in advanced stages of the disease, thus making the clinical diagnosis of the patients more reliable. Prospective studies of the diagnostic value of MR imaging in early degenerative parkinsonism are globally lacking and would seem an important research priority. In fact, it is in the early disease stages of parkinsonism when most diagnostic errors occur,[10,143,144,146] and where imaging or other diagnostic markers are most badly needed. Moreover, most of the studies have included only small patient numbers of on average 10 to 30 patients per disease entity, further limiting the generalization of the findings. Also, almost all MR imaging studies of PSP include patients suffering from the most reliably identifiable classic picture of PSP (ie, Richardson syndrome), whereas the true diagnostic dilemma lies with atypical presentations of PSP such as PSP-parkinsonism.[146–148] Given the pathologic heterogeneity of a "corticobasal syndrome," including CBD and other neurodegenerative causes such as PSP, Pick disease, and other frontotemporal lobar degenerations,[93,149] MR imaging studies of clinically defined CBD must also be discussed with a grain of caution.

Another major weakness of MR-based neuroimaging studies in parkinsonism in the past has been the heterogeneity of MR imaging protocols used, preventing compromising comparability between studies. Therefore, the definition of standardized protocols and algorithms in the performance of MR-based neuroimaging studies in parkinsonism represents a major issue in this research area, as reported previously for VBM studies.[40]

SUMMARY

Despite the aforementioned limitations, the different modern MR techniques have undoubtedly added to the differential diagnosis of neurodegenerative parkinsonism. Table 2 summarizes useful MR imaging findings to help clinicians diagnose patients presenting with parkinsonism. Only MR imaging findings that have been confirmed by at least 2 concordant studies are listed in Table 2. Even though cMR imaging still lacks sensitivity in distinguishing PD from MSA-P, PSP, and CBS, and also specificity in discriminating between the different APDs, it remains a useful tool for the exclusion of symptomatic causes of parkinsonism. Newer techniques including VBM, DW/DT imaging, or MT imaging raise hope for an increase in sensitivity for differential diagnostic issues, and have potential to provide insight into the pathophysiology of APD. Further prospective studies are required to determine whether these methods may yield added value for the clinical workup of patients. DW/DT imaging especially bears several advantages. DW/DT imaging may detect diffusion abnormalities in the basal ganglia and infratentorial structures in patients with APD at an early stage of disease. Furthermore, DW/DT imaging sequences are widely available on whole body MR scanners and can be acquired within a few minutes.

To determine which of the discussed techniques will emerge as standard investigation in the workup of PD and APD patients requires further prospective studies during early disease stages when the clinical diagnosis remains uncertain.

REFERENCES

1. Gilman S, Low PA, Quinn N, et al. Consensus statement on the diagnosis of multiple system atrophy. J Auton Nerv Syst 1998;74:189–92.
2. Gilman S, Wenning GK, Low PA, et al. Second consensus statement on the diagnosis of multiple system atrophy. Neurology 2008;71:670–6.
3. Hughes AJ, Ben-Shlomo Y, Daniel SE, et al. What features improve the accuracy of clinical diagnosis

in Parkinson's disease: a clinicopathologic study. Neurology 1992;42:1142–6.

4. Litvan I, Agid Y, Calne D, et al. Clinical research criteria for the diagnosis of progressive supranuclear palsy (Steele-Richardson-Olszewski syndrome): report of the NINDS-SPSP international workshop. Neurology 1996;47:1–9.

5. Litvan I, Bhatia KP, Burn DJ, et al. Movement Disorders Society Scientific Issues Committee report: SIC Task Force appraisal of clinical diagnostic criteria for parkinsonian disorders. Mov Disord 2003;18:467–86.

6. Hughes AJ, Daniel SE, Kilford L, et al. Accuracy of clinical diagnosis of idiopathic Parkinson's disease: a clinico-pathological study of 100 cases. J Neurol Neurosurg Psychiatr 1992;55:181–4.

7. Hughes AJ, Daniel SE, Ben-Shlomo Y, et al. The accuracy of diagnosis of parkinsonian syndromes in a specialist movement disorder service. Brain 2002;125:861–70.

8. Jankovic J, Rajput AH, McDermott MP, et al. The evolution of diagnosis in early Parkinson disease. Parkinson Study Group. Arch Neurol 2000;57:369–72.

9. Rajput AH, Rozdilsky B, Rajput A. Accuracy of clinical diagnosis in parkinsonism—a prospective study. Can J Neurol Sci 1991;18:275–8.

10. Tolosa E, Wenning G, Poewe W. The diagnosis of Parkinson's disease. Lancet Neurol 2006;5:75–86.

11. Dickson DW, Rademakers R, Hutton ML. Progressive supranuclear palsy: pathology and genetics. Brain Pathol 2007;17:74–82.

12. Lang AE, Lozano AM. Parkinson's disease. First of two parts. N Engl J Med 1998;339:1044–53.

13. Lang AE, Lozano AM. Parkinson's disease. Second of two parts. N Engl J Med 1998;339:1130–43.

14. Litvan I, Mangone CA, McKee A, et al. Natural history of progressive supranuclear palsy (Steele-Richardson-Olszewski syndrome) and clinical predictors of survival: a clinicopathological study. J Neurol Neurosurg Psychiatr 1996;60:615–20.

15. Marras C, Lang A. Invited article: changing concepts in Parkinson disease: moving beyond the decade of the brain. Neurology 2008;70:1996–2003.

16. Muller J, Wenning GK, Jellinger K, et al. Progression of Hoehn and Yahr stages in Parkinsonian disorders: a clinicopathologic study. Neurology 2000;55:888–91.

17. Rinne JO, Lee MS, Thompson PD, et al. Corticobasal degeneration. A clinical study of 36 cases. Brain 1994;117(Pt 5):1183–96.

18. Seppi K, Yekhlef F, Diem A, et al. Progression of parkinsonism in multiple system atrophy. J Neurol 2005;252:91–6.

19. Wenning GK, Ben SY, Magalhaes M, et al. Clinical features and natural history of multiple system atrophy. An analysis of 100 cases. Brain 1994;117(Pt 4):835–45.

20. Wenning GK, Colosimo C, Geser F, et al. Multiple system atrophy. Lancet Neurol 2004;3:93–103.

21. Dickersin K, Scherer R, Lefebvre C. Identifying relevant studies for systematic reviews. BMJ 1994;309:1286–91.

22. Drayer BP, Olanow W, Burger P, et al. Parkinson plus syndrome: diagnosis using high field MR imaging of brain iron. Radiology 1986;159:493–8.

23. Pastakia B, Polinsky R, Di CG, et al. Multiple system atrophy (Shy-Drager syndrome): MR imaging. Radiology 1986;159:499–502.

24. Farrall A. Magnetic resonance imaging: how to understand it. Pract Neurol 2006;6:318–25.

25. Duguid JR, De La PR, DeGroot J. Magnetic resonance imaging of the midbrain in Parkinson's disease. Ann Neurol 1986;20:744–7.

26. Gupta A, Dawson VL, Dawson TM. What causes cell death in Parkinson's disease? Ann Neurol 2008;64(Suppl 2):S3–15.

27. Hirsch EC, Hunot S. Neuroinflammation in Parkinson's disease: a target for neuroprotection? Lancet Neurol 2009;8:382–97.

28. Wilms H, Zecca L, Rosenstiel P, et al. Inflammation in Parkinson's diseases and other neurodegenerative diseases: cause and therapeutic implications. Curr Pharm Des 2007;13:1925–8.

29. Schwarz J, Weis S, Kraft E, et al. Signal changes on MRI and increases in reactive microgliosis, astrogliosis, and iron in the putamen of two patients with multiple system atrophy. J Neurol Neurosurg Psychiatr 1996;60:98–101.

30. Brass SD, Chen NK, Mulkern RV, et al. Magnetic resonance imaging of iron deposition in neurological disorders. Top Magn Reson Imaging 2006;17:31–40.

31. Haacke EM, Cheng NY, House MJ, et al. Imaging iron stores in the brain using magnetic resonance imaging. Magn Reson Imaging 2005;23:1–25.

32. Righini A, Antonini A, Ferrarini M, et al. Thin section MR study of the basal ganglia in the differential diagnosis between striatonigral degeneration and Parkinson disease. J Comput Assist Tomogr 2002;26:266–71.

33. Lee WH, Lee CC, Shyu WC, et al. Hyperintense putaminal rim sign is not a hallmark of multiple system atrophy at 3T. AJNR Am J Neuroradiol 2005;26:2238–42.

34. Brant-Zawadzki M, Gillan GD, Nitz WR. Mp Rage: a three-dimensional, T1-weighted, gradient-echo sequence—initial experience in the brain. Radiology 1992;182:769–75.

35. Hutchinson M, Raff U. Parkinson's disease: a novel MRI method for determining structural changes in

the substantia nigra. J Neurol Neurosurg Psychiatr 1999;67:815–8.

36. Hutchinson M, Raff U, Lebedev S. MRI correlates of pathology in parkinsonism: segmented inversion recovery ratio imaging (SIRRIM). Neuroimage 2003;20:1899–902.

37. Ashburner J, Friston KJ. Voxel-based morphometry—the methods. Neuroimage 2000;11:805–21.

38. Minnerop M, Specht K, Ruhlmann J, et al. Voxel-based morphometry and voxel-based relaxometry in multiple system atrophy—a comparison between clinical subtypes and correlations with clinical parameters. Neuroimage 2007;36:1086–95.

39. Specht K, Minnerop M, Muller-Hubenthal J, et al. Voxel-based analysis of multiple-system atrophy of cerebellar type: complementary results by combining voxel-based morphometry and voxel-based relaxometry. Neuroimage 2005;25:287–93.

40. Ridgway GR, Henley SM, Rohrer JD, et al. Ten simple rules for reporting voxel-based morphometry studies. Neuroimage 2008;40:1429–35.

41. Hagmann P, Jonasson L, Maeder P, et al. Understanding diffusion MR imaging techniques: from scalar diffusion-weighted imaging to diffusion tensor imaging and beyond. Radiographics 2006;26(Suppl 1):S205–23.

42. Le Bihan D. Looking into the functional architecture of the brain with diffusion MRI. Nat Rev Neurosci 2003;4:469–80.

43. Schocke MF, Seppi K, Esterhammer R, et al. Trace of diffusion tensor differentiates the Parkinson variant of multiple system atrophy and Parkinson's disease. Neuroimage 2004;21:1443–51.

44. Wolff SD, Balaban RS. Magnetization transfer contrast (MTC) and tissue water proton relaxation in vivo. Magn Reson Med 1989;10:135–44.

45. van Buchem MA, McGowan JC, Grossman RI. Magnetization transfer histogram methodology: its clinical and neuropsychological correlates. Neurology 1999;53:S23–8.

46. Fazekas F, Ropele S, Enzinger C, et al. MTI of white matter hyperintensities. Brain 2005;128:2926–32.

47. Trabesinger AH, Meier D, Boesiger P. In vivo ^{1}H NMR spectroscopy of individual human brain metabolites at moderate field strengths. Magn Reson Imaging 2003;21:1295–302.

48. Firbank MJ, Harrison RM, O'Brien JT. A comprehensive review of proton magnetic resonance spectroscopy studies in dementia and Parkinson's disease. Dement Geriatr Cogn Disord 2002;14:64–76.

49. Schocke MF, Berger T, Felber SR, et al. Serial contrast-enhanced magnetic resonance imaging and spectroscopic imaging of acute multiple sclerosis lesions under high-dose methylprednisolone therapy. Neuroimage 2003;20:1253–63.

50. Heiss WD, Hilker R. The sensitivity of 18-fluorodopa positron emission tomography and magnetic resonance imaging in Parkinson's disease. Eur J Neurol 2004;11:5–12.

51. Krauss JK, Paduch T, Mundinger F, et al. Parkinsonism and rest tremor secondary to supratentorial tumours sparing the basal ganglia. Acta Neurochir (Wien) 1995;133:22–9.

52. Manyam BV, Bhatt MH, Moore WD, et al. Bilateral striopallidodentate calcinosis: cerebrospinal fluid, imaging, and electrophysiological studies. Ann Neurol 1992;31:379–84.

53. Saatci I, Topcu M, Baltaoglu FF, et al. Cranial MR findings in Wilson's disease. Acta Radiol 1997;38:250–8.

54. Sibon I, Tison F. Vascular parkinsonism. Curr Opin Neurol 2004;17:49–54.

55. Tranchant C, Bhatia KP, Marsden CD. Movement disorders in multiple sclerosis. Mov Disord 1995;10:418–23.

56. McNeill A, Birchall D, Hayflick SJ, et al. T2* and FSE MRI distinguishes four subtypes of neurodegeneration with brain iron accumulation. Neurology 2008;70:1614–9.

57. Brooks DJ. Morphological and functional imaging studies on the diagnosis and progression of Parkinson's disease. J Neurol 2000;247(Suppl 2):II11–8.

58. Rutledge JN, Hilal SK, Silver AJ, et al. Study of movement disorders and brain iron by MR. AJR Am J Roentgenol 1987;149:365–79.

59. Savoiardo M, Girotti F, Strada L, et al. Magnetic resonance imaging in progressive supranuclear palsy and other parkinsonian disorders. J Neural Transm Suppl 1994;42:93–110.

60. Savoiardo M. Differential diagnosis of Parkinson's disease and atypical parkinsonian disorders by magnetic resonance imaging. Neurol Sci 2003;24(Suppl 1):S35–7.

61. Hu MT, White SJ, Herlihy AH, et al. A comparison of (18)F-dopa PET and inversion recovery MRI in the diagnosis of Parkinson's disease. Neurology 2001;56:1195–200.

62. Minati L, Grisoli M, Carella F, et al. Imaging degeneration of the substantia nigra in Parkinson disease with inversion-recovery MR imaging. AJNR Am J Neuroradiol 2007;28:309–13.

63. Seppi K, Schocke MF. An update on conventional and advanced magnetic resonance imaging techniques in the differential diagnosis of neurodegenerative parkinsonism. Curr Opin Neurol 2005;18:370–5.

64. Schrag A, Kingsley D, Phatouros C, et al. Clinical usefulness of magnetic resonance imaging in multiple system atrophy. J Neurol Neurosurg Psychiatr 1998;65:65–71.

65. Schrag A, Rinne JO, Burn DJ, et al. Olivopontocerebellar atrophy and multiple system atrophy:

clinical follow-up of 10 patients studied with PET. Ann Neurol 1998;44:151–2.

66. Abe K, Hikita T, Yokoe M, et al. The "cross" signs in patients with multiple system atrophy: a quantitative study. J Neuroimaging 2006;16:73–7.

67. Kraft E, Schwarz J, Trenkwalder C, et al. The combination of hypointense and hyperintense signal changes on T2-weighted magnetic resonance imaging sequences: a specific marker of multiple system atrophy? Arch Neurol 1999;56:225–8.

68. Bhattacharya K, Saadia D, Eisenkraft B, et al. Brain magnetic resonance imaging in multiple-system atrophy and Parkinson disease: a diagnostic algorithm. Arch Neurol 2002;59:835–42.

69. Ito S, Shirai W, Hattori T. Evaluating posterolateral linearization of the putaminal margin with magnetic resonance imaging to diagnose the Parkinson variant of multiple system atrophy. Mov Disord 2007;22:578–81.

70. Schocke MF, Seppi K, Esterhammer R, et al. Diffusion-weighted MRI differentiates the Parkinson variant of multiple system atrophy from PD. Neurology 2002;58:575–80.

71. Seppi K, Schocke MF, Mair KJ, et al. Progression of putaminal degeneration in multiple system atrophy: a serial diffusion MR study. Neuroimage 2006;31:240–5.

72. Yekhlef F, Ballan G, Macia F, et al. Routine MRI for the differential diagnosis of Parkinson's disease, MSA, PSP, and CBD. J Neural Transm 2003;110:151–69.

73. Horimoto Y, Aiba I, Yasuda T, et al. Longitudinal MRI study of multiple system atrophy—when do the findings appear, and what is the course? J Neurol 2002;249:847–54.

74. Lee EA, Cho HI, Kim SS, et al. Comparison of magnetic resonance imaging in subtypes of multiple system atrophy. Parkinsonism Relat Disord 2004;10:363–8.

75. Watanabe H, Saito Y, Terao S, et al. Progression and prognosis in multiple system atrophy: an analysis of 230 Japanese patients. Brain 2002;125:1070–83.

76. Kraft E, Trenkwalder C, Auer DP. T2*-weighted MRI differentiates multiple system atrophy from Parkinson's disease. Neurology 2002;59:1265–7.

77. von Lewinski F, Werner C, Jorn T, et al. T2*-weighted MRI in diagnosis of multiple system atrophy. A practical approach for clinicians. J Neurol 2007;254:1184–8.

78. Barsottini OG, Ferraz HB, Maia AC Jr, et al. Differentiation of Parkinson's disease and progressive supranuclear palsy with magnetic resonance imaging: the first Brazilian experience. Parkinsonism Relat Disord 2007;13:389–93.

79. Oba H, Yagishita A, Terada H, et al. New and reliable MRI diagnosis for progressive supranuclear palsy. Neurology 2005;64:2050–5.

80. Paviour DC, Price SL, Stevens JM, et al. Quantitative MRI measurement of superior cerebellar peduncle in progressive supranuclear palsy. Neurology 2005;64:675–9.

81. Paviour DC, Price SL, Jahanshahi M, et al. Regional brain volumes distinguish PSP, MSA-P, and PD: MRI-based clinico-radiological correlations. Mov Disord 2006;21:989–96.

82. Paviour DC, Price SL, Jahanshahi M, et al. Longitudinal MRI in progressive supranuclear palsy and multiple system atrophy: rates and regions of atrophy. Brain 2006;129:1040–9.

83. Schrag A, Good CD, Miszkiel K, et al. Differentiation of atypical parkinsonian syndromes with routine MRI. Neurology 2000;54:697–702.

84. Slowinski J, Imamura A, Uitti RJ, et al. MR imaging of brainstem atrophy in progressive supranuclear palsy. J Neurol 2008;255:37–44.

85. Soliveri P, Monza D, Paridi D, et al. Cognitive and magnetic resonance imaging aspects of corticobasal degeneration and progressive supranuclear palsy. Neurology 1999;53:502–7.

86. Sitburana O, Ondo WG. Brain magnetic resonance imaging (MRI) in parkinsonian disorders. Parkinsonism Relat Disord 2009;15:165–74.

87. Righini A, Antonini A, De NR, et al. MR imaging of the superior profile of the midbrain: differential diagnosis between progressive supranuclear palsy and Parkinson disease. AJNR Am J Neuroradiol 2004;25:927–32.

88. Warmuth-Metz M, Naumann M, Csoti I, et al. Measurement of the midbrain diameter on routine magnetic resonance imaging: a simple and accurate method of differentiating between Parkinson disease and progressive supranuclear palsy. Arch Neurol 2001;58:1076–9.

89. Graber JJ, Staudinger R. Teaching NeuroImages: "Penguin" or "hummingbird" sign and midbrain atrophy in progressive supranuclear palsy. Neurology 2009;72:e81.

90. Kato N, Arai K, Hattori T. Study of the rostral midbrain atrophy in progressive supranuclear palsy. J Neurol Sci 2003;210:57–60.

91. Kataoka H, Tonomura Y, Taoka T, et al. Signal changes of superior cerebellar peduncle on fluid-attenuated inversion recovery in progressive supranuclear palsy. Parkinsonism Relat Disord 2008;14:63–5.

92. Hauser RA, Murtaugh FR, Akhter K, et al. Magnetic resonance imaging of corticobasal degeneration. J Neuroimaging 1996;6:222–6.

93. Josephs KA, Tang-Wai DF, Edland SD, et al. Correlation between antemortem magnetic resonance imaging findings and pathologically confirmed corticobasal degeneration. Arch Neurol 2004;61:1881–4.

94. Nicoletti G, Fera F, Condino F, et al. MR imaging of middle cerebellar peduncle width: differentiation of

multiple system atrophy from Parkinson disease. Radiology 2006;239:825–30.

95. Quattrone A, Nicoletti G, Messina D, et al. MR imaging index for differentiation of progressive supranuclear palsy from Parkinson disease and the Parkinson variant of multiple system atrophy. Radiology 2008;246:214–21.

96. Cosottini M, Ceravolo R, Faggioni L, et al. Assessment of midbrain atrophy in patients with progressive supranuclear palsy with routine magnetic resonance imaging. Acta Neurol Scand 2007;116: 37–42.

97. Cordato NJ, Pantelis C, Halliday GM, et al. Frontal atrophy correlates with behavioural changes in progressive supranuclear palsy. Brain 2002;125: 789–800.

98. Ghaemi M, Hilker R, Rudolf J, et al. Differentiating multiple system atrophy from Parkinson's disease: contribution of striatal and midbrain MRI volumetry and multi-tracer PET imaging. J Neurol Neurosurg Psychiatr 2002;73:517–23.

99. Groschel K, Hauser TK, Luft A, et al. Magnetic resonance imaging-based volumetry differentiates progressive supranuclear palsy from corticobasal degeneration. Neuroimage 2004;21:714–24.

100. Schulz JB, Skalej M, Wedekind D, et al. Magnetic resonance imaging-based volumetry differentiates idiopathic Parkinson's syndrome from multiple system atrophy and progressive supranuclear palsy. Ann Neurol 1999;45:65–74.

101. Camicioli R. Identification of parkinsonism and Parkinson's disease. Drugs Today (Barc) 2002;38:677–86.

102. Jokinen P, Bruck A, Aalto S, et al. Impaired cognitive performance in Parkinson's disease is related to caudate dopaminergic hypofunction and hippocampal atrophy. Parkinsonism Relat Disord 2009; 15:88–93.

103. Laakso MP, Partanen K, Riekkinen P, et al. Hippocampal volumes in Alzheimer's disease, Parkinson's disease with and without dementia, and in vascular dementia: An MRI study. Neurology 1996;46:678–81.

104. Burton EJ, McKeith IG, Burn DJ, et al. Cerebral atrophy in Parkinson's disease with and without dementia: a comparison with Alzheimer's disease, dementia with Lewy bodies and controls. Brain 2004;127:791–800.

105. Nagano-Saito A, Washimi Y, Arahata Y, et al. Cerebral atrophy and its relation to cognitive impairment in Parkinson disease. Neurology 2005;64:224–9.

106. Summerfield C, Junque C, Tolosa E, et al. Structural brain changes in Parkinson disease with dementia: a voxel-based morphometry study. Arch Neurol 2005;62:281–5.

107. Brenneis C, Seppi K, Schocke MF, et al. Voxel-based morphometry detects cortical atrophy in the Parkinson variant of multiple system atrophy. Mov Disord 2003;18:1132–8.

108. Brenneis C, Boesch SM, Egger KE, et al. Cortical atrophy in the cerebellar variant of multiple system atrophy: a voxel-based morphometry study. Mov Disord 2006;21:159–65.

109. Specht K, Minnerop M, Abele M, et al. In vivo voxel-based morphometry in multiple system atrophy of the cerebellar type. Arch Neurol 2003;60:1431–5.

110. Brenneis C, Egger K, Scherfler C, et al. Progression of brain atrophy in multiple system atrophy. A longitudinal VBM study. J Neurol 2007;254:191–6.

111. Brenneis C, Seppi K, Schocke M, et al. Voxel based morphometry reveals a distinct pattern of frontal atrophy in progressive supranuclear palsy. J Neurol Neurosurg Psychiatr 2004;75:246–9.

112. Price S, Paviour D, Scahill R, et al. Voxel-based morphometry detects patterns of atrophy that help differentiate progressive supranuclear palsy and Parkinson's disease. Neuroimage 2004;23:663–9.

113. Boxer AL, Geschwind MD, Belfor N, et al. Patterns of brain atrophy that differentiate corticobasal degeneration syndrome from progressive supranuclear palsy. Arch Neurol 2006;63:81–6.

114. Blain CR, Barker GJ, Jarosz JM, et al. Measuring brain stem and cerebellar damage in parkinsonian syndromes using diffusion tensor MRI. Neurology 2006;67:2199–205.

115. Paviour DC, Thornton JS, Lees AJ, et al. Diffusion-weighted magnetic resonance imaging differentiates parkinsonian variant of multiple-system atrophy from progressive supranuclear palsy. Mov Disord 2007;22:68–74.

116. Rizzo G, Martinelli P, Manners D, et al. Diffusion-weighted brain imaging study of patients with clinical diagnosis of corticobasal degeneration, progressive supranuclear palsy and Parkinson's disease. Brain 2008;131:2690–700.

117. Seppi K, Schocke MF, Esterhammer R, et al. Diffusion-weighted imaging discriminates progressive supranuclear palsy from PD, but not from the Parkinson variant of multiple system atrophy. Neurology 2003;60:922–7.

118. Seppi K, Schocke MF, Donnemiller E, et al. Comparison of diffusion-weighted imaging and [123I]IBZM-SPECT for the differentiation of patients with the Parkinson variant of multiple system atrophy from those with Parkinson's disease. Mov Disord 2004;19:1438–45.

119. Chan LL, Rumpel H, Yap K, et al. Case control study of diffusion tensor imaging in Parkinson's disease. J Neurol Neurosurg Psychiatr 2007;78:1383–6.

120. Yoshikawa K, Nakata Y, Yamada K, et al. Early pathological changes in the parkinsonian brain demonstrated by diffusion tensor MRI. J Neurol Neurosurg Psychiatr 2004;75:481–4.

121. Vaillancourt DE, Spraker MB, Prodoehl J, et al. High-resolution diffusion tensor imaging in the substantia nigra of de novo Parkinson disease. Neurology 2009;72:1378–84.

122. Karagulle Kendi AT, Lehericy S, Luciana M, et al. Altered diffusion in the frontal lobe in Parkinson disease. AJNR Am J Neuroradiol 2008;29:501–5.

123. Tessa C, Giannelli M, Della NR, et al. A whole-brain analysis in de novo Parkinson disease. AJNR Am J Neuroradiol 2008;29:674–80.

124. Scherfler C, Seppi K, Donnemiller E, et al. Voxel-wise analysis of [123I]beta-CIT SPECT differentiates the Parkinson variant of multiple system atrophy from idiopathic Parkinson's disease. Brain 2005; 128:1605–12.

125. Ito M, Watanabe H, Kawai Y, et al. Usefulness of combined fractional anisotropy and apparent diffusion coefficient values for detection of involvement in multiple system atrophy. J Neurol Neurosurg Psychiatr 2007;78:722–8.

126. Kollensperger M, Seppi K, Liener C, et al. Diffusion weighted imaging best discriminates PD from MSA-P: a comparison with tilt table testing and heart MIBG scintigraphy. Mov Disord 2007;22:1771–6.

127. Pellecchia MT, Barone P, Mollica C, et al. Diffusion-weighted imaging in multiple system atrophy: a comparison between clinical subtypes. Mov Disord 2009;24:689–96.

128. Nicoletti G, Lodi R, Condino F, et al. Apparent diffusion coefficient measurements of the middle cerebellar peduncle differentiate the Parkinson variant of MSA from Parkinson's disease and progressive supranuclear palsy. Brain 2006;129:2679–87.

129. Seppi K, Schocke MF, Prennschuetz-Schuetzenau K, et al. Topography of putaminal degeneration in multiple system atrophy: a diffusion magnetic resonance study. Mov Disord 2006;21:847–52.

130. Nicoletti G, Tonon C, Lodi R, et al. Apparent diffusion coefficient of the superior cerebellar peduncle differentiates progressive supranuclear palsy from Parkinson's disease. Mov Disord 2008;23:2370–6.

131. Kanazawa M, Shimohata T, Terajima K, et al. Quantitative evaluation of brainstem involvement in multiple system atrophy by diffusion-weighted MR imaging. J Neurol 2004;251:1121–4.

132. Boelmans K, Kaufmann J, Bodammer N, et al. Involvement of motor pathways in corticobasal syndrome detected by diffusion tensor tractography. Mov Disord 2009;24:168–75.

133. Anik Y, Iseri P, Demirci A, et al. Magnetization transfer ratio in early period of Parkinson disease. Acad Radiol 2007;14:189–92.

134. Eckert T, Sailer M, Kaufmann J, et al. Differentiation of idiopathic Parkinson's disease, multiple system atrophy, progressive supranuclear palsy, and healthy controls using magnetization transfer imaging. Neuroimage 2004;21:229–35.

135. Tambasco N, Pelliccioli GP, Chiarini P, et al. Magnetization transfer changes of grey and white matter in Parkinson's disease. Neuroradiology 2003;45:224–30.

136. Chaudhuri KR, Lemmens GM, Williams SC, et al. Proton magnetic resonance spectroscopy of the striatum in Parkinson's disease patients with motor response fluctuations. Parkinsonism Relat Disord 1996;2:63–7.

137. Clarke CE, Lowry M. Systematic review of proton magnetic resonance spectroscopy of the striatum in Parkinsonian syndromes. Eur J Neurol 2001;8:573–7.

138. Davie CA, Wenning GK, Barker GJ, et al. Differentiation of multiple system atrophy from idiopathic Parkinson's disease using proton magnetic resonance spectroscopy. Ann Neurol 1995;37:204–10.

139. Federico F, Simone IL, Lucivero V, et al. Proton magnetic resonance spectroscopy in Parkinson's disease and atypical parkinsonian disorders. Mov Disord 1997;12:903–9.

140. Federico F, Simone IL, Lucivero V, et al. Proton magnetic resonance spectroscopy in Parkinson's disease and progressive supranuclear palsy. J Neurol Neurosurg Psychiatr 1997;62:239–42.

141. Federico F, Simone IL, Lucivero V, et al. Usefulness of proton magnetic resonance spectroscopy in differentiating parkinsonian syndromes. Ital J Neurol Sci 1999;20:223–9.

142. Watanabe H, Fukatsu H, Katsuno M, et al. Multiple regional ^{1}H-MR spectroscopy in multiple system atrophy: NAA/Cr reduction in pontine base as a valuable diagnostic marker. J Neurol Neurosurg Psychiatr 2004;75:103–9.

143. Osaki Y, Wenning GK, Daniel SE, et al. Do published criteria improve clinical diagnostic accuracy in multiple system atrophy? Neurology 2002;59:1486–91.

144. Osaki Y, Ben-Shlomo Y, Lees AJ, et al. Accuracy of clinical diagnosis of progressive supranuclear palsy. Mov Disord 2004;19:181–9.

145. Schrag A, Ben-Shlomo Y, Quinn N. How valid is the clinical diagnosis of Parkinson's disease in the community? J Neurol Neurosurg Psychiatr 2002;73:529–34.

146. Williams DR, Lees AJ. How do patients with parkinsonism present? A clinicopathological study. Intern Med J 2009;39:7–12.

147. Williams DR, de SR, Paviour DC, et al. Characteristics of two distinct clinical phenotypes in pathologically proven progressive supranuclear palsy: Richardson's syndrome and PSP-parkinsonism. Brain 2005;128:1247–58.

148. Williams DR, Lees AJ, Wherrett JR, et al. J. Clifford Richardson and 50 years of progressive supranuclear palsy. Neurology 2008;70:566–73.

149. Wadia PM, Lang AE. The many faces of cortico-basal degeneration. Parkinsonism Relat Disord 2007;13(Suppl 3):S336–40.

150. Shiga K, Yamada K, Yoshikawa K, et al. Local tissue anisotropy decreases in cerebellopetal fibers and pyramidal tract in multiple system atrophy. J Neurol 2005;252:589–96.

151. Padovani A, Borroni B, Brambati SM, et al. Diffusion tensor imaging and voxel based morphometry study in early progressive supranuclear palsy. J Neurol Neurosurg Psychiatr 2006;77:457–63.

152. Nilsson C, Markenroth BK, Brockstedt S, et al. Tracking the neurodegeneration of parkinsonian disorders—a pilot study. Neuroradiology 2007;49:111–9.

153. Tir M, Delmaire C, le TV, et al. Motor-related circuit dysfunction in MSA-P: usefulness of combined whole-brain imaging analysis. Mov Disord 2009; 24:863–70.

Extrapyramidal Syndromes: PET and SPECT

Klaus Tatsch, MD

KEYWORDS

- Parkinsonism • Differential diagnosis • PET/SPECT
- Dopaminergic system • Sympathetic innervation
- Glucose metabolism

Extrapyramidal syndromes (ES) belong to the most common neurologic illnesses. Because new and promising therapeutic options are currently under development, there is a substantial demand for molecular imaging procedures with the potential to identify the pathologic changes of those illnesses. This article gives an overview of the current positron emission tomography (PET) and single photon emission computed tomography (SPECT) applications for diagnosing ES and focuses on their use in clinical practice.

Among ES, the parkinsonian syndromes (PS) play a predominant role. This syndromatic umbrella term comprises 3 etiologically different entities: Parkinson disease (PD; idiopathic parkinsonian syndrome), atypical parkinsonian syndromes (aPS; parkinsonian syndromes caused by other neurodegenerative diseases), and symptomatic (secondary) parkinsonism (sPS), including some other major differential diagnoses.[1] The group of aPS includes multiple system atrophies (MSAs, parkinsonian and cerebellar type), progressive supranuclear palsy (PSP), corticobasal degeneration (CBD), and spinocerebellar ataxias (SCAs). Dementia with Lewy bodies (DLB), presumably reflecting a different variant of PD, also plays an increasing role. The sPS group includes vascular-, drug-, toxic-, metabolic-, and inflammatory-induced parkinsonism, normal pressure hydrocephalus, and, more rarely, cases of injury- or tumor-induced parkinsonism. Clinically, ET is

the most important differential diagnosis in this group, when compared with PD and aPS.

The diagnosis of PS is usually established by using well-defined clinical criteria. Particularly in the early stages of disease, if clinical findings are subtle, mono-symptomatic (eg, isolated tremor), or equivocal, it may be difficult to establish the correct diagnosis. In the past various publications have addressed the issue of misdiagnosis from different points of view.[2–7]

In patients suffering from PS, establishing an early and accurate diagnosis has an impact on their management, helps to avoid wrong treatment decisions, and may aid in selecting patients for therapeutic trials with newly developed drugs. Clinically, PS are characterized by disturbances in motor function ,such as tremor, rigidity, bradykinesia, and postural abnormalities. Conventional structural imaging with CT and MRI has limited value in the early diagnosis of PS, because, in many instances, structural abnormalities may only be present in more advanced disease or may be difficult to assess in individual subjects. Conversely, molecular imaging with PET and SPECT offers various tools for the classification and differential diagnosis of PS. Apart from the assessment of brain perfusion, glucose metabolism, and cardiac sympathetic denervation, nuclear medicine techniques allow the imaging of key functions of neurotransmission involved in the etiology of neurodegenerative PS. Here, the

Department of Nuclear Medicine, Municipal Hospital Karlsruhe Inc, Moltkestrasse 90, D-76133 Karlsruhe, Germany
E-mail address: klaus.tatsch@klinikum-karlsruhe.de

Neuroimag Clin N Am 20 (2010) 57–68
doi:10.1016/j.nic.2009.08.017

dopaminergic system plays a dominant role in clinical routine assessment.[8-15]

IMAGING TECHNIQUES

Since pathology in neurodegenerative PS involves the dopaminergic pathway, PET and SPECT investigations of the pathway deliver important diagnostic contributions. Presynaptic nigrostriatal terminal function can be assessed with radioligands suitable for imaging at least 3 different functions: the aromatic amino acid decarboxylase activity (PET: fluorodopa)[9,10]; the vesicular monoamine transporter type 2 (VMAT2, PET: dihydrotetrabenazine),[16] and the plasma membrane dopamine transporter (DAT, PET and SPECT: cocaine analogs).[8] Imaging of postsynaptic dopamine receptors has focused on the D_2-like receptor system (PET: raclopride, desmethoxyfallypride[DMFP]; SPECT: iodobenzamide, iodobenzofuran, epidepride).[8,13,15] The dopaminergic synapse and dopaminergic neurotransmission are schematically illustrated in **Fig. 1**, highlighting the more widely used PET and SPECT tracers targeting these systems. Apart from the dopaminergic system, other approaches like assessment of brain glucose metabolism[17] or cardiac sympathetic denervation of the heart (PET: hydroxyephedrine [HED], SPECT: metaiodobenzylguanidine

[MIBG])[18,19] may also aid in the further classification of PS.

CHARACTERISTIC PET AND SPECT FINDINGS IN PS

Clinicians seek answers to the following key questions: (1) whether the patient suffers from neurodegenerative PS or from a different (non-neurodegenerative) disease; (2) if neurodegenerative PS is likely, whether PD or aPS is the most probable diagnosis; and (3) if the latter is diagnosed, the aPS category.

The following sections briefly summarize major findings reported for the most frequent PS and provide a helpful scheme for answering the questions raised by the use of nuclear imaging techniques.

NEURODEGENERATIVE PARKINSONIAN SYNDROMES
PD

The predominant pathology in PD, which accounts for about 70% to 80% of PS, is the loss of dopaminergic neurons that project from the substantia nigra pars compacta in the midbrain to the striatum (putamen and caudate nucleus). The loss of neurons results in a dopaminergic deficit, which is believed to contribute to the clinical symptoms. Typically, the projections to the posterior putamen are affected earlier and to a greater extent than those to the caudate. The clinical diagnosis of PD relies on the presence of cardinal motor features and a favorable response to dopaminergic medication. However, because PD shares some major features with several other disorders, there is evidence that clinically established diagnoses may be wrong in early- and even late-stage disease.[2-5,7] When the diagnosis is unclear, neuroimaging with PET or SPECT may help clarify it.

The biochemical hallmark of PD is the degeneration of the presynaptic nigrostriatal nerve fibers, whereas the postsynaptic side bearing the receptors remains intact, at least initially. Imaging of presynaptic terminal functions, therefore, reveals reduced radioligand uptake in the striatum of PD patients with a more pronounced decrease in the (posterior) putamen than in the caudate, and, usually, also reveals an asymmetry with more severe affection of the striatum contralateral to the limbs that are more affected, clinically.[8-10,13] Significant correlations between disease severity and disability stages with the extent of the reduction of presynaptic terminal measures have been reported.[20-22] In addition, studies in patients with early PD and those with hemi-PD (Hoehn and

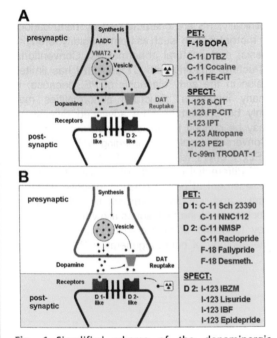

Fig. 1. Simplified scheme of the dopaminergic synapse and the dopaminergic neurotransmission illustrating the pre- (*A*) and postsynaptic (*B*) targets for frequently used PET and SPECT ligands.

Yahr stage I) have concordantly shown a bilateral deficit in dopamine function. These findings were not only observed in the striatum and especially the putamen corresponding to the symptomatic limbs but also in the contralateral putamen associated with the still asymptomatic side of the body.[23–25] These results strongly suggest that the aforementioned imaging techniques are capable of discriminating between subjects with early PD and healthy ones and that may also be suitable for detecting preclinical disease in sporadic and familial PD.[26–30] Additionally, longitudinal imaging studies have highlighted their role in determining intraindividual disease progression.[23,31–35] The annual rate of decline of the respective outcome measure in PD patients has been shown to range from 5% to 13% in patients with early-stage PD, whereas in those with longer disease duration, the annual decline of presynaptic outcome measures was lower (approximately 2% to 3%). In atypical PS, annual progression seems much faster; for example, in MSA patients, values of around 15% per year have been reported.[36,37] Imaging of presynaptic functions has also been used in clinical trials as endpoint measures of potential disease-modifying therapies. Fluorodopa PET and 2β-carbomethoxy-3β-(4-iodophenyl)-N-(3-fluoropropyl) nortropane (ß-CIT) SPECT studies have demonstrated that the respective outcome measure showed a milder decline in patients receiving therapy with a dopamine agonist compared with levodopa.[38–40] These trial results evoked an intense and somewhat controversial discussion on whether these imaging modalities may serve as useful surrogate markers for proving potential neuroprotective effects of newly developed drugs.[41–43]

PET and SPECT with D_2-receptor antagonists have also been extensively used to study the postsynaptic striatal D_2-receptor availability of patients with PD.[8,10,13,15] At least in earlier stages of the disease, uniformly elevated D_2-receptor binding has been reported in the striatum contralateral to the more affected limb. Characteristically, in these cases, binding is higher in the putamen than in the caudate, and even higher in the posterior than in the anterior putamen (Fig. 2). This upregulation has been interpreted as the brain's attempt to compensate for the dopaminergic deficit related to the presynaptic nerve cell loss and may be considered characteristic of PD; whereas in aPS, the postsynaptic side is also affected by neurodegeneration and displays reduced D_2-receptor density.

Some recent clinical trials using PET and SPECT imaging have found that a distinct subgroup of subjects with clinical criteria for (early-stage) PD presented with normal scans. These patients have been termed SWEDDs (subjects with scans without evidence of dopaminergic deficit). To date, SWEDDs have been mentioned in at least 3 large-scale clinical trials, the CALM-PD-CIT trial, the ELLDOPA study, and the REAL-PET study.[38–40] Combining the data of these trials suggests that SWEDDs may be present in about 11% of included subjects (45 of 410 clinically diagnosed PD cases). This number is consistent with reported rates in the clinical literature of misdiagnosis of early-stage PD by movement disorder specialists. One possible and self-evident conclusion, therefore, would be that SWEDDs may simply reflect clinically misdiagnosed PD patients. Furthermore, follow-up data have shown that SWEDDs maintain the feature of noncompromised presynaptic functions over time and, thus, clearly differ from typical PD subjects. SWEDDs, therefore, may represent a distinct population within the mentioned clinical trials, and whether these subjects have PD or an alternative diagnosis has been questioned. Histopathologic diagnosis obtained in SWEDDs might be the clue to unravel their mystery; unfortunately it is still unavailable.

APS

MSA

MSA is a sporadic progressive neurodegenerative disorder that may account for up to 10% of patients with ES. Clinically, MSA is characterized by varying degrees of parkinsonism, cerebellar ataxia, and autonomic dysfunction. In terms of dependency of the predominant phenotype of the motor disorder, MSA is mainly classified into a parkinsonian type (MSA-P) and a cerebellar type (MSA-C). Pathologic studies exhibit neuronal degeneration and gliosis in the basal ganglia, brainstem, cerebellum, and spinal cord. In MSA, annual progression seems much faster compared with PD; annual loss in striatal binding around 15% per year has been reported. Because MSA is characterized by a degeneration of the pre- and postsynaptic dopaminergic system, PET and SPECT investigations of both show reduced binding (Fig. 3).[15,44–47] The major difference compared to PD, therefore, is the presence of pathologic findings on the postsynaptic level, which allows one to distinguish between MSA and PD. On the presynaptic level, reliable differential diagnosis between MSA and PD is not possible.

PSP

PSP is a rapidly progressing degenerative disease belonging to the family of tauopathies. Clinically, it is characterized by parkinsonism with

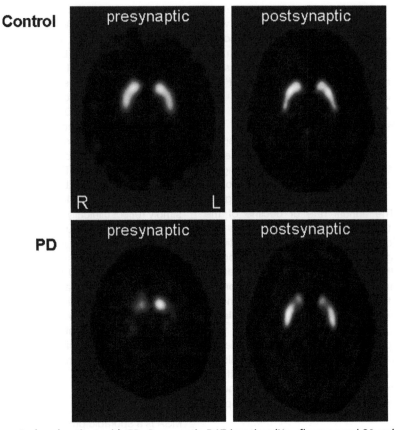

Fig. 2. Healthy control and patient with PD. Presynaptic DAT imaging (N-ω-fluoropropyl-2β-carbomethoxy-3β-(4-iodophenyl)nortropane [FP-CIT] SPECT) clearly reveals reduced striatal binding in the PD patient with more severe affection of the (posterior) putamen and an asymmetry with disadvantage to the right side, which is contralateral to the predominant clinical findings (left sided). Postsynaptic D_2-receptors (DMFP PET) show preserved and upregulated binding, which is more accentuated in the posterior putamen compared with the anterior putamen and the caudate. Note the asymmetry with higher binding in the right striatum, which is inversely related to the more severe presynaptic deficit at this location.

bradykinesia and rigidity, postural instability, and a pseudobulbar syndrome with dysarthria and dysphagia. The key feature of PSP, the supranuclear palsy of vertical gaze is rarely present at onset and usually appears later. Histopathologic findings show cell loss, gliosis, and accumulation of tau proteins in different brain regions, such as brainstem and basal ganglia, with the cortex being usually spared. Because neurodegeneration in PSP also affects the pre- and postsynaptic dopaminergic system, the PET and SPECT findings are similar to those in MSA subjects, showing a marked reduction on pre- and postsynaptic levels. Therefore, PSP patients cannot be reliably distinguished with pre- nor postsynaptic tracers from those with MSA. However, pathologic PET and SPECT findings on the postsynaptic level allow one to discriminate between PSP and PD.[15,44,45,48]

CBD

CBD is an asymmetric, progressive, neurodegenerative disease characterized by cortical and subcortical involvement, with motor and cognitive dysfunction. Patients with CBD often present initially with apraxia and parkinsonian symptoms (akinetic rigid type), which usually do not respond to dopaminergic therapy. Dystonia and alien limb phenomenon are also frequently observed symptoms. Pathology reveals an asymmetric frontoparietal neuronal loss and gliosis, nigral degeneration, and variable subcortical involvement. Because corticobasal ganglionic degeneration involves the striatal presynaptic and possibly also the postsynaptic dopaminergic system, PET and SPECT studies of the latter should present with pathologic results. Concordantly, reduction in striatal fluorodopa uptake has been described and SPECT studies have also revealed a marked decrease in

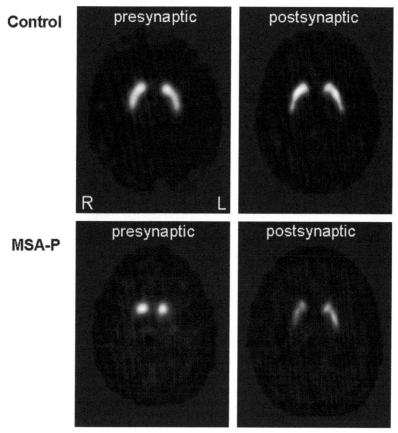

Fig. 3. Healthy control and patient with MSA. Presynaptic DAT(FP-CIT SPECT) and postsynaptic D_2-receptor images (DMFP PET) concordantly show reduced binding of the respective tracers, both with more severe affection of the right side. The pathologic imaging results reflect degeneration of both pre- and postsynaptic fibers of the dopaminergic system within the striatum. Note that presynaptic imaging alone cannot reliably distinguish between PD (see Fig. 2) and MSA (as an example of aPS). Only at the postsynaptic level is there a marked difference between PD (no neurodegeneration) and aPS (neurodegeneration).

dopamine transporter binding.[45,49,50] Generally, a clear asymmetry is noted with predominant affection of the striatum contralateral to clinical symptoms. Both caudate and putamen seem to be similarly affected. Reports on the postsynaptic receptor status in CBD are more rare and somewhat controversial, describing preserved and diminished striatal binding.[49]

Other Neurodegenerative Extrapyramidal Syndromes

SCAs are a genetically heterogeneous group of autosomal dominant ataxias, which may present as pure cerebellar and various noncerebellar syndromes including parkinsonism. Imaging studies have shown decreased glucose metabolism in the cerebellum and various parts of the cerebral cortex, depending on the SCA subtypes. Decreased presynaptic dopaminergic terminal function

has been reported in SCA2 and SCA3[51–54] and there are also some preliminary reports on reduced postsynaptic D_2-receptor binding potential.[51,55] Huntington disease (HD) is an autosomal dominant neurodegenerative disorder and clinically characterized by progressive cognitive impairment, neuropsychiatric symptoms, and abnormalities of movement including chorea and akinetic rigidity. Histopathologically, HD is characterized by neuronal loss and gliosis in the striatum. Accordingly PET and SPECT studies show substantial decrease in striatal perfusion, glucose metabolism, and severely compromised pre- and postsynaptic dopaminergic functions.[46,56–61] Wilson disease (WD) is also a genetically determined disorder (autosomal recessive) that is characterized by a deficiency of biliary copper excretion resulting in pathologic copper deposition in various organs including the brain. WD goes along with extrapyramidal symptoms including parkinsonism. Similar to HD, patients with WD also present with compromised binding to pre- and postsynaptic dopaminergic targets in the striatum and show reduced striatal metabolism and perfusion, apart from the concomitant involvement of other brain areas.[62–67] HD and WD are generally diagnosed clinically and genetically, with the role of functional imaging being restricted to scientific applications.

Differential Diagnosis of the Common Neurodegenerative PS

For the differential diagnosis of PD versus aPS, various nuclear medicine techniques may be applied.

As already mentioned, postsynaptic D_2-like receptor imaging is useful in distinguishing between PD and aPS, with the former showing preserved receptors and the latter, compromised binding because of degeneration of postsynaptic fibers.[8,9,11,13,15] A representative case example is shown in **Figs. 2** and **3**. As optimized by receiver operating characteristic (ROC) analyses, reported sensitivities and specificities were 87% and 73%, respectively for SPECT and 89% and 86%, respectively for PET investigations.[68,69] Combining the information of pre- and postsynaptic dopaminergic imaging marginally increased diagnostic accuracy compared with postsynaptic imaging alone.[68] Even though reasonable results are delivered for distinguishing PD from aPS, these imaging techniques fail to further distinguish between different types of aPS reliably.

Another molecular imaging approach for distinguishing PD from aPS addresses the sympathetic denervation of the heart, rather than focusing on the brain.[18,19,70–74] For this purpose, HED and MIBG may be used as PET and SPECT tracers, respectively. Autonomic abnormalities in PD have been ascribed to postganglionic sympathetic nerve dysfunction, which is depicted by the mentioned imaging techniques. In this respect, patients with PD behave differently from those with aPS, in whom normal or only mild reduction of cardiac uptake is present. Pathologically, aPS goes along with a central and preganglionic denervation that is not targeted by the mentioned tracers. Based on this principle, a reasonable number of studies have used this type of cardiac imaging for the differential diagnosis of PD and aPS. However, the diagnostic accuracy of this approach has been criticized.[72] Overlapping values in cardiac binding of both groups raised concerns regarding the use of these techniques as the sole method for diagnostic discrimination.[19] Limitations and confounders of the methods have to be taken into account (eg, sympathetic denervation related to other diseases, such as diabetes mellitus or several cardiac diseases).

A third option for distinguishing PD from aPS is based on the pattern analysis of brain glucose metabolism. This is the only approach that also allows one to distinguish between the various aPS. By using modern processing tools like anatomical standardization with pixelwise evaluation or discriminant and network analyses, typical metabolic patterns may be identified, which result in high diagnostic accuracies.[17,75] A recent study assessing PD, MSA, PSP, and CBD on a single-case basis reported sensitivities between 85% and 96% and specificities between 60% and 92%.[17] The study used statistical parametric mapping to create disease-related templates in which regional features were determined and used for defining or supporting specific diseases. Briefly, hypermetabolism of the dorsolateral putamen was considered indicative of PD, bilateral hypometabolism of the putamen and cerebellum, of MSA, hypometabolism of brain stem and midline frontal cortex, of PSP, and asymmetric hypometabolism of basal ganglia and some cortical areas, of CBD.

SYMPTOMATIC PARKINSONIAN SYNDROMES

One important question for clinicians is whether patients with equivocal or unclear symptoms suffer from neurodegenerative PS or symptomatic PS that are not associated with degeneration of striatal dopaminergic terminals. Whereas assessment of glucose metabolism or regional cerebral blood flow is of little help in diagnosing sPS, imaging of presynaptic terminal function has been shown to be highly accurate for exclusion of nigrostriatal degeneration. Patients with drug-induced or psychogenic parkinsonism, with ET and other tremor syndromes, with normal pressure hydrocephalus, or with dopa-responsive dystonia, all show preserved dopamine terminals and thus, can be reliably distinguished from PD and aPS.[14,76–80] Some examples are shown in **Fig. 4**.

The role of vascular parkinsonism (VP) in this context is still indeterminate. Diagnosis of VP is often established clinically in conjunction with the results of morphologic imaging, which has provided circumstantial support for the concept of VP, together with histopathologic evidence supporting small vessel disease as a cause of VP. Based on clinical and histopathologic findings, 2 types of VP can be identified, one with insidious onset and vascular lesions diffusely located in the watershed areas (VPi) and another with acute onset and strategic infarcts in areas involved in the striato-thalamo-cortical circuit (VPa). A recent study described a significant presynaptic

PET and SPECT images of presynaptic dopaminergic functions inform on the number and integrity of nigrostriatal terminals

Neurodegenerative PS

Parkinson's Disease (PD)

Familial PD

Atypical Parkinsonian Syndromes
  PSP, MSA, CBD,
  Lewy Body Disease,
  Huntington's Disease
  Wilson's Disease

Diseases without presynaptic deficit

Symptomatic PS
  psychogenic, drug induced

Pseudo-PS
  NPH, vascular PS (?)

Tremor Syndromes
  Essential Tremor (ET),
  psychogenic, drug induced

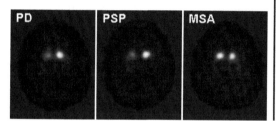 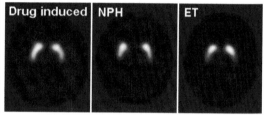

Fig. 4. Presynaptic imaging can be used reliably to confirm or exclude neurodegenerative PS. If binding is normal, presence of sPS is highly likely. Apart from drug-induced or psychogenic PS and normal pressure hydrocephalus, tremor syndromes play an important role in this category, particularly, ET. In all these diseases, images of presynaptic terminal functions show normal striatal binding, thus indicating absence of neurodegenerative parkinsonism (*right*).

dopaminergic deficit in patients with VPi and VPa compared with controls.[81] The image pattern was similar to the one observed in PD, except that the asymmetry index comparing right-to-left striatal binding was lower than in PD, suggesting more symmetrical involvement in VP, and in particular VPi subjects. This is consistent with the notion that disease in the vascular group is more diffusely distributed (as also supported by the evidence of diffuse small vessel disease on MRI images) than in PD. In some patients with VPa, "punched out" striatal uptake was seen, corresponding to areas of focal infarction. Understandably, in those cases, striatal asymmetry was more marked. In general, data in the literature do not consistently report on deficits of presynaptic functions in VP or on normal or near-normal findings.[82] These inconsistencies suggest that VP may be a heterogeneous group with subtypes or stages in which presynaptic functions may be preserved.

DLB

Neurodegenerative dementia is an increasingly common disorder, with Alzheimer disease (AD) and DLB accounting for most cases. Unfortunately, some overlap in clinical presentations among both may lead to diagnostic confusion.[6,83] On the other hand, accurate clinical detection is important for drug treatment, because a considerable number of patients with DLB show good responsiveness to cholinesterase inhibitors but extreme sensitivity to side effects of neuroleptic drugs. Clinical features aiding in the diagnosis of DLB and AD have shown an acceptable high specificity (>90%) for the diagnosis of DLB, but at an unacceptable low sensitivity (mean: 49%, range 0%–83%). Thus, there is a need to improve the diagnosis of DLB in vivo.

Several studies have addressed the changes in cerebral perfusion and glucose metabolism in neurodegenerative dementias, and distinct patterns have been suggested to identify and distinguish between various types.[84–86] The methodology has improved over the years, and more refined data analysis has been established as routine procedure, for example, based on voxelwise comparison with normal databases after stereotactic normalization. Another highly accurate instrument has been added, addressing

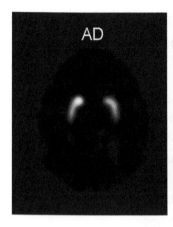 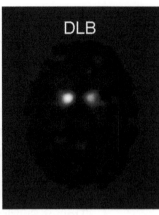

Fig. 5. Differential diagnosis between DLB and AD. Subjects with DLB present with clearly reduced binding to presynaptic dopaminergic markers (*right*). In this respect images are hardly distinguishable from PD or aPS (compare also Figs. 2–4). In contrast, patients with AD present with no or only marginal reduction of these functions (*left*), thus allowing a reliable separation between DLB and AD subjects.

a striking biological difference between DLB and AD, which is the severe nigrostriatal degeneration and consequent loss of presynaptic dopaminergic terminal functions that occurs in DLB but not to any significant extent in AD (Fig. 5). This notion is substantiated by concordant antemortem and postmortem findings. Autoradiographic studies have proven the distinguishability of DLB from AD based on presynaptic dopaminergic markers,[87,88] and single-site[89–91] and multicenter studies[92] have shown that DLB and AD can be distinguished at high accuracy levels during life, independent of the technology used (SPECT or PET) and the target addressed (dopamine turnover, DAT, or VMAT2). In the studies that report numbers, the sensitivities and specificities relating to clinical diagnoses based on the established consensus criteria ranged from 78% to 86% and 85% to 100%, respectively.[90,92,93] Imaging findings correlated even better with those at autopsy (sensitivity: 88%, specificity: 100%).[94] Corresponding data for imaging postsynaptic dopamine receptors are comparatively rare and less conclusive, and thus suggest a limited role for this purpose. Presynaptic measures may be extended by adding complementary information derived from other imaging techniques. Combining 2 parameters from different studies, such as fluorodeoxyglucose (FDG) and dihydrotetrabenazine for assessment of metabolic abnormalities in conjunction with nigrostriatal dopaminergic function may improve discrimination between groups of patients with dementia.[95]

SUMMARY

Molecular imaging with PET and SPECT provides valuable diagnostic information that is complementary to the clinical, genetic, and electrophysiological routine workup of patients with extrapyramidal syndromes. Imaging delivers

results with high diagnostic accuracy and therefore, has impact on individual therapeutic strategies and appraisal of the corresponding prognosis. For confirmation of neurodegenerative parkinsonism (PD and aPS) or its exclusion (sPS), assessment of presynaptic dopaminergic terminal function is suggested as the most appropriate method. If binding is normal, sPS is highly likely. Clinically, ET is probably the most important differential diagnosis in this group. If presynaptic binding is compromised and thus indicates the presence of a neurodegenerative PS, postsynaptic D_2-receptor imaging allows one to further distinguish between PD and aPS. Alternatively, for the same purpose, imaging of the cardiac sympathetic denervation might be used, but with care, respecting its limitations. If either approach points to an aPS, FDG PET may allow one to further distinguish between the important entities in this group (MSA, PSP, and CBD), based on distinct metabolic patterns indicative of each of these diseases. For the differential diagnosis between DLB and AD, assessment of presynaptic dopaminergic terminal function may be suggested as an easy and reliable approach.

REFERENCES

1. Leitlinie: Parkinson-syndrome: diagnostik und therapie. überarbeitete Auflage. In: Leitlinien für diagnostik und therapie in der neurologie. 4th edition. Stuttgart: Georg Thieme Verlag; 2008.
2. Catafau AM, Tolosa E. Impact of dopamine transporter SPECT using 123I-Ioflupane on diagnosis and management of patients with clinically uncertain Parkinsonian syndromes. Mov Disord 2004;19: 1175–82.
3. Hughes AJ, Ben-Shlomo Y, Daniel SE, et al. What features improve the accuracy of clinical diagnosis in Parkinson's disease: a clinicopathologic study. 1992. Neurology 2001;57:S34–8.

4. Hughes AJ, Daniel SE, Kilford L, et al. Accuracy of clinical diagnosis of idiopathic Parkinson's disease: a clinico-pathological study of 100 cases. J Neurol Neurosurg Psychiatr 1992;55:181–4.

5. Marshall VL, Reininger CB, Marquardt M, et al. Parkinson's disease is overdiagnosed clinically at baseline in diagnostically uncertain cases: a 3-year European multicenter study with repeat [123I]FP-CIT SPECT. Mov Disord 2009;24:500–8.

6. McKeith I, Mintzer J, Aarsland D, et al. Dementia with Lewy bodies. Lancet Neurol 2004;3:19–28.

7. Meara J, Bhowmick BK, Hobson P. Accuracy of diagnosis in patients with presumed Parkinson's disease. Age Ageing 1999;28:99–102.

8. Booij J, Tissingh G, Winogrodzka A, et al. Imaging of the dopaminergic neurotransmission system using single-photon emission tomography and positron emission tomography in patients with parkinsonism. Eur J Nucl Med 1999;26:171–82.

9. Brooks DJ. Assessment of Parkinson's disease with imaging. Parkinsonism Relat Disord 2007;13(Suppl 3):S268–75.

10. Brooks DJ. Neuroimaging in Parkinson's disease. NeuroRx 2004;1:243–54.

11. Brucke T, Djamshidian S, Bencsits G, et al. SPECT and PET imaging of the dopaminergic system in Parkinson's disease. J Neurol 2000;247(Suppl 4):IV/2–7.

12. Marshall V, Grosset D. Role of dopamine transporter imaging in routine clinical practice. Mov Disord 2003;18:1415–25.

13. Nikolaus S, Antke C, Kley K, et al. Investigating the dopaminergic synapse in vivo. I. Molecular imaging studies in humans. Rev Neurosci 2007;18:439–72.

14. Scherfler C, Schwarz J, Antonini A, et al. Role of DAT-SPECT in the diagnostic work up of parkinsonism. Mov Disord 2007;22:1229–38.

15. Tatsch K. Imaging of the dopaminergic system in parkinsonism with SPET. Nucl Med Commun 2001; 22:819–27.

16. Frey KA, Koeppe RA, Kilbourn MR. Imaging the vesicular monoamine transporter. Adv Neurol 2001; 86:237–47.

17. Eckert T, Barnes A, Dhawan V, et al. FDG PET in the differential diagnosis of parkinsonian disorders. Neuroimage 2005;26:912–21.

18. Post KK, Singer C, Papapetropoulos S. Cardiac denervation and dysautonomia in Parkinson's disease: a review of screening techniques. Parkinsonism Relat Disord 2008;14:524–31.

19. Raffel DM, Koeppe RA, Little R, et al. PET measurement of cardiac and nigrostriatal denervation in Parkinsonian syndromes. J Nucl Med 2006;47:1769–77.

20. Rinne JO, Ruottinen H, Bergman J, et al. Usefulness of a dopamine transporter PET ligand [(18)F]beta-CFT in assessing disability in Parkinson's disease. J Neurol Neurosurg Psychiatr 1999;67:737–41.

21. Seibyl JP, Marek KL, Quinlan D, et al. Decreased single-photon emission computed tomographic [123I]beta-CIT striatal uptake correlates with symptom severity in Parkinson's disease. Ann Neurol 1995;38:589–98.

22. Tatsch K, Schwarz J, Mozley PD, et al. Relationship between clinical features of Parkinson's disease and presynaptic dopamine transporter binding assessed with [123I]IPT and single-photon emission tomography. Eur J Nucl Med 1997;24:415–21.

23. Brooks DJ. Morphological and functional imaging studies on the diagnosis and progression of Parkinson's disease. J Neurol 2000;247(Suppl 2):II11–8.

24. Marek KL, Seibyl JP, Zoghbi SS, et al. [123I] beta-CIT/SPECT imaging demonstrates bilateral loss of dopamine transporters in hemi-Parkinson's disease. Neurology 1996;46:231–7.

25. Winogrodzka A, Bergmans P, Booij J, et al. [(123)I]beta-CIT SPECT is a useful method for monitoring dopaminergic degeneration in early stage Parkinson's disease. J Neurol Neurosurg Psychiatr 2003;74:294–8.

26. Berendse HW, Booij J, Francot CM, et al. Subclinical dopaminergic dysfunction in asymptomatic Parkinson's disease patients' relatives with a decreased sense of smell. Ann Neurol 2001;50:34–41.

27. Khan NL, Brooks DJ, Pavese N, et al. Progression of nigrostriatal dysfunction in a parkin kindred: an [18F]dopa PET and clinical study. Brain 2002; 125(Pt 10):2248–56.

28. Laihinen A, Ruottinen H, Rinne JO, et al. Risk for Parkinson's disease: twin studies for the detection of asymptomatic subjects using [18F]6-fluorodopa PET. J Neurol 2000;247(Suppl 2):II110–3.

29. Piccini P, Morrish PK, Turjanski N, et al. Dopaminergic function in familial Parkinson's disease: a clinical and 18F-dopa positron emission tomography study. Ann Neurol 1997;41:222–9.

30. Wolters EC, Francot C, Bergmans P, et al. Preclinical (premotor) Parkinson's disease. J Neurol 2000; 247(Suppl 2):II103–9.

31. Morrish PK, Rakshi JS, Bailey DL, et al. Measuring the rate of progression and estimating the preclinical period of Parkinson's disease with [18F]dopa PET. J Neurol Neurosurg Psychiatr 1998;64:314–9.

32. Nurmi E, Bergman J, Eskola O, et al. Progression of dopaminergic hypofunction in striatal subregions in Parkinson's disease using [18F]CFT PET. Synapse 2003;48:109–15.

33. Nurmi E, Ruottinen HM, Bergman J, et al. Rate of progression in Parkinson's disease: a 6-[18F]fluoro-L-dopa PET study. Mov Disord 2001;16:608–15.

34. Schwarz J, Storch A, Koch W, et al. Loss of dopamine transporter binding in Parkinson's disease follows a single exponential rather than linear decline. J Nucl Med 2004;45:1694–7.

35. Stoffers D, Booij J, Bosscher L, et al. Early-stage [123I]beta-CIT SPECT and long-term clinical follow-up in patients with an initial diagnosis of Parkinson's disease. Eur J Nucl Med Mol Imaging 2005;32:689–95.

36. Pirker W, Djamshidian S, Asenbaum S, et al. Progression of dopaminergic degeneration in Parkinson's disease and atypical parkinsonism: a longitudinal beta-CIT SPECT study. Mov Disord 2002;17:45–53.

37. Pirker W, Holler I, Gerschlager W, et al. Measuring the rate of progression of Parkinson's disease over a 5-year period with beta-CIT SPECT. Mov Disord 2003;18:1266–72.

38. Fahn S, Oakes D, Shoulson I, et al. Levodopa and the progression of Parkinson's disease. N Engl J Med 2004;351:2498–508.

39. Parkinson Study Group. Dopamine transporter brain imaging to assess the effects of pramipexole vs levodopa on Parkinson disease progression. JAMA 2002;287:1653–61.

40. Whone AL, Watts RL, Stoessl AJ, et al. Slower progression of Parkinson's disease with ropinirole versus levodopa: the REAL-PET study. Ann Neurol 2003;54:93–101.

41. Marek K, Jennings D, Seibyl J. Dopamine agonists and Parkinson's disease progression: what can we learn from neuroimaging studies. Ann Neurol 2003; 53(Suppl 3):S160–6 [discussion: S166–9].

42. Morrish PK. How valid is dopamine transporter imaging as a surrogate marker in research trials in Parkinson's disease? Mov Disord 2003;18(Suppl 7):S63–70.

43. Seibyl J, Jennings D, Tabamo R, et al. Unique roles of SPET brain imaging in clinical and research studies. Lessons from Parkinson's disease research. Q J Nucl Med Mol Imaging 2005;49:215–21.

44. Brucke T, Asenbaum S, Pirker W, et al. Measurement of the dopaminergic degeneration in Parkinson's disease with [123I] beta-CIT and SPECT. Correlation with clinical findings and comparison with multiple system atrophy and progressive supranuclear palsy. J Neural Transm Suppl 1997;50:9–24.

45. Pirker W, Asenbaum S, Bencsits G, et al. [123I]beta-CIT SPECT in multiple system atrophy, progressive supranuclear palsy, and corticobasal degeneration. Mov Disord 2000;15:1158–67.

46. Pirker W, Asenbaum S, Wenger S, et al. Iodine-123-epidepride-SPECT: studies in Parkinson's disease, multiple system atrophy and Huntington's disease. J Nucl Med 1997;38:1711–7.

47. Varrone A, Marek KL, Jennings D, et al. [(123)I]beta-CIT SPECT imaging demonstrates reduced density of striatal dopamine transporters in Parkinson's disease and multiple system atrophy. Mov Disord 2001;16:1023–32.

48. Seppi K, Scherfler C, Donnemiller E, et al. Topography of dopamine transporter availability in progressive supranuclear palsy: a voxelwise [123I]beta-CIT SPECT analysis. Arch Neurol 2006; 63:1154–60.

49. Klaffke S, Kuhn AA, Plotkin M, et al. Dopamine transporters, D2 receptors, and glucose metabolism in corticobasal degeneration. Mov Disord 2006;21:1724–7.

50. Laureys S, Salmon E, Garraux G, et al. Fluorodopa uptake and glucose metabolism in early stages of corticobasal degeneration. J Neurol 1999;246: 1151–8.

51. Boesch SM, Donnemiller E, Muller J, et al. Abnormalities of dopaminergic neurotransmission in SCA2: a combined 123I-betaCIT and 123I-IBZM SPECT study. Mov Disord 2004;19:1320–5.

52. Varrone A, Salvatore E, De Michele G, et al. Reduced striatal [123 I]FP-CIT binding in SCA2 patients without parkinsonism. Ann Neurol 2004;55: 426–30.

53. Wang PS, Liu RS, Yang BH, et al. Regional patterns of cerebral glucose metabolism in spinocerebellar ataxia type 2, 3 and 6: a voxel-based FDG-positron emission tomography analysis. J Neurol 2007;254: 838–45.

54. Wullner U, Reimold M, Abele M, et al. Dopamine transporter positron emission tomography in spinocerebellar ataxias type 1, 2, 3, and 6. Arch Neurol 2005;62:1280–5.

55. Reimold M, Globas C, Gleichmann M, et al. Spinocerebellar ataxia type 1, 2, and 3 and restless legs syndrome: striatal dopamine D2 receptor status investigated by [11C]raclopride positron emission tomography. Mov Disord 2006;21:1667–73.

56. Andrews TC, Brooks DJ. Advances in the understanding of early Huntington's disease using the functional imaging techniques of PET and SPET. Mol Med Today 1998;4:532–9.

57. Boecker H, Kuwert T, Langen KJ, et al. SPECT with HMPAO compared to PET with FDG in Huntington disease. J Comput Assist Tomogr 1994;18:542–8.

58. Ichise M, Toyama H, Fornazzari L, et al. Iodine-123-IBZM dopamine D2 receptor and technetium-99m-HMPAO brain perfusion SPECT in the evaluation of patients with and subjects at risk for Huntington's disease. J Nucl Med 1993;34: 1274–81.

59. Leblhuber F, Brucker B, Reisecker F, et al. Single photon emission computed tomography in subjects at risk for Huntington's chorea. J Neurol 1990;237: 496–8.

60. Leblhuber F, Hoell K, Reisecker F, et al. Single photon emission computed tomography in Huntington's chorea. Psychiatry Res 1989;29:337–9.

61. Leslie WD, Greenberg CR, Abrams DN, et al. Clinical deficits in Huntington disease correlate with reduced striatal uptake on iodine-123 epidepride single-photon emission tomography. Eur J Nucl Med 1999;26:1458–64.

62. Barthel H, Hermann W, Kluge R, et al. Concordant pre- and postsynaptic deficits of dopaminergic neurotransmission in neurologic Wilson disease. AJNR Am J Neuroradiol 2003;24:234–8.

63. Jeon B, Kim JM, Jeong JM, et al. Dopamine transporter imaging with [123I]-beta-CIT demonstrates presynaptic nigrostriatal dopaminergic damage in Wilson's disease. J Neurol Neurosurg Psychiatr 1998;65:60–4.

64. Oder W, Brucke T, Kollegger H, et al. Dopamine D2 receptor binding is reduced in Wilson's disease: correlation of neurological deficits with striatal 123I-iodobenzamide binding. J Neural Transm 1996;103:1093–103.

65. Oertel WH, Tatsch K, Schwarz J, et al. Decrease of D2 receptors indicated by 123I-iodobenzamide single-photon emission computed tomography relates to neurological deficit in treated Wilson's disease. Ann Neurol 1992;32:743–8.

66. Tatsch K, Schwarz J, Oertel WH, et al. SPECT imaging of dopamine D2 receptors with 123I-IBZM: initial experience in controls and patients with Parkinson's syndrome and Wilson's disease. Nucl Med Commun 1991;12:699–707.

67. Wang P, Hu P, Yue DC, et al. The clinical value of Tc-99m TRODAT-1 SPECT for evaluating disease severity in young patients with symptomatic and asymptomatic Wilson disease. Clin Nucl Med 2007;32:844–9.

68. Koch W, Hamann C, Radau PE, et al. Does combined imaging of the pre- and postsynaptic dopaminergic system increase the diagnostic accuracy in the differential diagnosis of parkinsonism? Eur J Nucl Med Mol Imaging 2007;34:1265–73.

69. Tatsch K, Wängler B, Bötzel K, et al. Differential diagnosis of parkinsonism with [F-18]DMFP PET. J Nucl Med 2008;49(Suppl 1):5P.

70. Nagayama H, Hamamoto M, Ueda M, et al. Reliability of MIBG myocardial scintigraphy in the diagnosis of Parkinson's disease. J Neurol Neurosurg Psychiatr 2005;76:249–51.

71. Saiki S, Hirose G, Sakai K, et al. Cardiac 123I-MIBG scintigraphy can assess the disease severity and phenotype of PD. J Neurol Sci 2004;220:105–77.

72. Sawada H, Oeda T, Yamamoto K, et al. Diagnostic accuracy of cardiac metaiodobenzylguanidine scintigraphy in Parkinson disease. Eur J Neurol 2009;16:174–82.

73. Spiegel J, Hellwig D, Farmakis G, et al. Myocardial sympathetic degeneration correlates with clinical phenotype of Parkinson's disease. Mov Disord 2007;22:1004–8.

74. Spiegel J, Mollers MO, Jost WH, et al. FP-CIT and MIBG scintigraphy in early Parkinson's disease. Mov Disord 2005;20:552–61.

75. Van Laere K, Casteels C, De Ceuninck L, et al. Dual-tracer dopamine transporter and perfusion SPECT in differential diagnosis of parkinsonism using template-based discriminant analysis. J Nucl Med 2006;47:384–92.

76. Asenbaum S, Pirker W, Angelberger P, et al. [123I]beta-CIT and SPECT in essential tremor and Parkinson's disease. J Neural Transm 1998;105:1213–28.

77. Benamer TS, Patterson J, Grosset DG, et al. Accurate differentiation of parkinsonism and essential tremor using visual assessment of [123I]-FP-CIT SPECT imaging: the [123I]-FP-CIT study group. Mov Disord 2000;15:503–10.

78. Booij J, Speelman JD, Horstink MW, et al. The clinical benefit of imaging striatal dopamine transporters with [123I]FP-CIT SPET in differentiating patients with presynaptic parkinsonism from those with other forms of parkinsonism. Eur J Nucl Med 2001;28:266–72.

79. Huang CC, Yen TC, Weng YH, et al. Normal dopamine transporter binding in dopa responsive dystonia. J Neurol 2002;249:1016–20.

80. Jeon BS, Jeong JM, Park SS, et al. Dopamine transporter density measured by [123I]beta-CIT single-photon emission computed tomography is normal in dopa-responsive dystonia. Ann Neurol 1998;43:792–800.

81. Zijlmans JC, Daniel SE, Hughes AJ, et al. Clinicopathological investigation of vascular parkinsonism, including clinical criteria for diagnosis. Mov Disord 2004;19:630–40.

82. Gerschlager W, Bencsits G, Pirker W, et al. [123I]beta-CIT SPECT distinguishes vascular parkinsonism from Parkinson's disease. Mov Disord 2002;17:518–23.

83. Tatsch K. Imaging of the dopaminergic system in differential diagnosis of dementia. Eur J Nucl Med Mol Imaging 2008;35(Suppl 1):S51–7.

84. Herholz K, Carter SF, Jones M. Positron emission tomography imaging in dementia. Br J Radiol 2007;80(Spec No 2):S160–7.

85. Silverman DH. Brain 18F-FDG PET in the diagnosis of neurodegenerative dementias: comparison with perfusion SPECT and with clinical evaluations lacking nuclear imaging. J Nucl Med 2004;45:594–607.

86. Van Heertum RL, Tikofsky RS. Positron emission tomography and single-photon emission computed tomography brain imaging in the evaluation of dementia. Semin Nucl Med 2003;33:77–85.

87. Piggott MA, Marshall EF, Thomas N, et al. Striatal dopaminergic markers in dementia with Lewy bodies, Alzheimer's and Parkinson's diseases: rostrocaudal distribution. Brain 1999;122(Pt 8):1449–68.

88. Suzuki M, Desmond TJ, Albin RL, et al. Striatal monoaminergic terminals in Lewy body and Alzheimer's dementias. Ann Neurol 2002;51:767–71.

89. Koeppe RA, Gilman S, Junck L, et al. Differentiating Alzheimer's disease from dementia with Lewy

bodies and Parkinson's disease with (+)-[11C]dihy-drotetrabenazine positron emission tomography. Alzheimers Dement 2008;4(1 Suppl 1):S67–76.

90. O'Brien JT, Colloby S, Fenwick J, et al. Dopamine transporter loss visualized with FP-CIT SPECT in the differential diagnosis of dementia with Lewy bodies. Arch Neurol 2004;61:919–25.

91. Walker Z, Costa DC, Walker RW, et al. Differentiation of dementia with Lewy bodies from Alzheimer's disease using a dopaminergic presynaptic ligand. J Neurol Neurosurg Psychiatr 2002;73:134–40.

92. McKeith I, O'Brien J, Walker Z, et al. Sensitivity and specificity of dopamine transporter imaging with 123I-FP-CIT SPECT in dementia with Lewy bodies: a phase III, multicentre study. Lancet Neurol 2007; 6:305–13.

93. Walker Z, Costa DC, Walker RW, et al. Striatal dopamine transporter in dementia with Lewy bodies and Parkinson disease: a comparison. Neurology 2004; 62:1568–72.

94. Walker Z, Jaros E, Walker RW, et al. Dementia with Lewy bodies: a comparison of clinical diagnosis, FP-CIT single photon emission computed tomography imaging and autopsy. J Neurol Neurosurg Psychiatr 2007;78:1176–81.

95. Koeppe RA, Gilman S, Joshi A, et al. 11C-DTBZ and 18F-FDG PET measures in differentiating dementias. J Nucl Med 2005;46:936–44.

The Role of Imaging in the Diagnosis of Vascular Parkinsonism

Jan C.M. Zijlmans, MD, PhD

KEYWORDS

• Vascular parkinsonism • MRI • CT • SPECT • Diagnosis

PARKINSONISM

Parkinsonism is a syndrome that features bradykinesia (slowness of the initiation of voluntary movement) and at least 1 of the following conditions: rest tremor, muscular rigidity, or postural instability. In 1929, Critchley[1] identified a type of parkinsonism caused by cerebrovascular disease in his report on "arteriosclerotic parkinsonism." It required the development of computed tomography (CT) and magnetic resonance imaging (MRI) 50 years later to find evidence for Critchley's ideas and what is now commonly known as vascular parkinsonism (VP).[2–6] Ischemic vascular lesions that may lead to VP are lacunar infarctions, white matter hyperintensities, and less common large vessel infarctions. A comparison of 5 different European studies showed a prevalence rate of 3% of VP.[7] In case the onset of parkinsonism was associated with a cerebrovascular event, VP was diagnosed. Probably the real prevalence is higher because only few patients with VP have an acute onset.[6,8]

CLINICAL FEATURES

In the classical type of VP, as reported by Thompson and Marsden[4] and FitzGerald and Jankovic,[5] difficulty in walking is the most important initial symptom. Therefore, the classical type is also called lower-half[4] or lower-body parkinsonism.[5] In patients suffering from the classical type, the gait is disordered by shuffling, short steps, variable base (narrow to wide), start and turn hesitation, and moderate disequilibrium. In addition, the arm swing in patients with VP is usually more preserved than in patients with Parkinson disease (PD).[4,5,9]

Depending on their onset, 2 types of VP can be distinguished[6]: one with an insidious onset and its vascular lesions diffusely located in the watershed areas (VPi) and the other with an acute onset and lesions located in the subcortical gray nuclei (striatum, globus pallidus, and thalamus) (VPa). Winikates and Jankovic[8] later confirmed the 2 different types of onset. In about one-quarter of the patients with VP, the symptoms start acutely.[6,8]

CLINICAL DIAGNOSIS

Winikates and Jankovic[8] categorized patients with parkinsonism and a vascular score of 2 or more on a rating scale as having VP. In this way, many patients with PD and vascular risk factors can be misdiagnosed as having VP. Criteria for the clinical diagnosis of VP have been proposed, which are derived from a postmortem examination study.[10] See **Box 1** for the criteria for clinical diagnosis of VP.

ETIOLOGY

In the "classical clinical type" of VP, parkinsonism is attributed to diffuse periventricular and frontal white matter damage[4] because similar clinical features occur in normal pressure hydrocephalus and in some cases of frontal parasagittal meningioma, in which the same structures are compromised. According to Thompson and Marsden,[4] disconnection of thalamocortical fibers to the supplementary motor area and cerebellar fibers

Department of Neurology, Amphia Hospital, Molengracht 21, 4818 CK, Breda, The Netherlands
E-mail address: jzijlmans@amphia.nl

Neuroimag Clin N Am 20 (2010) 69–76
doi:10.1016/j.nic.2009.08.006

a. Parkinsonism

bradykinesia (slowness of initiation of voluntary movement with progressive reduction in speed and amplitude of repetitive actions in either upper limb or lower limb, including the presence of reduced step length) and at least 1 of the following:

rest tremor, muscular rigidity, or postural instability not caused by primary visual, vestibular, cerebellar or proprioceptive dysfunction

b. Cerebrovascular disease

- evidence of relevant cerebrovascular disease by brain imaging (CT or MRI) or
- the presence of focal signs or symptoms that are consistent with stroke.

c. A relationship between these 2 disorders. In practice

- an acute or delayed progressive onset with infarcts in or near areas that can increase the basal ganglia motor output (GPe [globus pallidus pars external] or SNc [substantia nigra pars compacta]) or decrease the thalamocortical drive directly (VL[ventral lateral] nuclei of the thalamus, large frontal lobe infarct). At onset, parkinsonism consists of a contralateral bradykinetic rigid syndrome or shuffling gait within 1 year after a stroke (VPa).
- an insidious onset of parkinsonism with extensive subcortical white matter lesions, bilateral symptoms at onset, and the presence of early shuffling gait or early cognitive dysfunction (VPi); the "classical clinical type."

Exclusion criteria

- a history of repeated head injury
- encephalitis
- neuroleptic treatment at onset of symptoms
- the presence of cerebral tumor or communicating hydrocephalus
- other alternative explanation for Parkinson syndrome

thalamocortical drive to premotor areas and also subsequent development of parkinsonism. According to many previous publications, parkinsonism is also attributed to strategic infarcts in the basal ganglia or thalamus. A causal relationship between strategic infarcts and parkinsonism is reported only in a few publications that described the cases in which the onset is (sub) acute or accompanied by other symptoms of a stroke related to the same lesion.[2,3,6,8,12–24] Lesions in specific areas that theoretically can cause parkinsonism (GPe, VL/VA of thalamus, and SNc) have been described by a few investigators.[2,16,18,21–23] The infarct is located in the hemisphere or brainstem contralateral to parkinsonism in most cases in which a vascular cause is acceptable and a single lesion is seen in the basal ganglia or thalamus.[12,14–18,20–22,24]

PATHOPHYSIOLOGY

The most supported hypothesis about the pathogenesis of subcortical lesions was originally proposed by Binswanger and Alzheimer.[25,26] They suggested that the white matter softening can be attributed to subcortical ischemia as a result of arteriolosclerosis of the long penetrating arteries. According to this view, arteriolosclerosis of long penetrating arteries that are poorly provided with collateral anastomoses can result in ischemia of the distal fields of these vessels, that is, periventricularly and in the watershed zones. Transient episodes of hypotension caused by excessive antihypertensive medication or heart failure[27] and hyperviscosity[28] may provoke or aggravate white matter disease in an already compromised cerebral blood flow.[29,30] The typically hypertensive changes of small vessel disease can occasionally be found in a patient who is not hypertensive or diabetic.[31] Conversely, not every elderly patient with hypertension develops small vessel disease.[32] These points suggest that factors other than hypertension and diabetes, such as a cerebrovascular accident, cardiac disease, or carotid pathology, are probably also involved in the development of hypertensive arteriolopathy.[33] Many investigators stated that the clinical significance of subcortical lesions depends on the severity and location of lesions.[6,32,34] A threshold extent of subcortical lesions may be necessary before symptoms appear.[6,34,35]

DIFFERENTIAL DIAGNOSIS

Features that are usually considered to favor a diagnosis of idiopathic PD[36] are also frequently present in VP and include micrographia,

to the leg area is the underlying mechanism that causes the gait disorder in VP.

In accordance with current concepts of putamenal efferents directed toward the basal ganglia output nuclei,[11] one might expect that vascular lesions in the SNc (substantia nigra pars compacta), GPe (globus pallidus pars externa), or the VA (ventral anterior)/VL (ventral lateral) nuclei of the thalamus induce decreased cogwheeling, stooped posture, facial masking, hypophonia, and a positive response to levodopa. However, application of the more stringent UK Parkinson's Disease Society Brain Bank criteria for the diagnosis of idiopathic PD[37] excludes this diagnosis in most patients with VP. In case a slowly progressive gait disorder presents itself with a shuffling gait, then a normal pressure hydrocephalus or a frontal lobe tumor must be considered. A clinical diagnosis together with a radiologic diagnosis of probable multiple system atrophy,[38] progressive supranuclear palsy (PSP),[39] or dementia with Lewy bodies[40] probably excludes a diagnosis of VP in most cases.[10] Dubinsky and Jankovic[41] and Winikates and Jankovic[42] suggested the presence of a particular subtype of VP that they called vascular PSP. In one report, the brains of 2 patients with vascular PSP showed (besides the common diffuse white matter lesions) additional lesions in the dorsal pons and in the thalamus.

Brain Imaging

In the last century, CT and MRI were mainly used to exclude hydrocephalus, mass lesions, or subdural hematomas in atypical parkinsonism. They now can support the clinical diagnosis of VP with positive imaging findings. One has to consider the 2 different locations of lesions with their related types of onset: an insidious onset type presenting itself with white matter lesions that are diffusely located in the watershed areas and an acute onset type with lesions located in contralateral strategic areas (globus pallidus,

thalamus, substantia nigra, and frontal lobe). MRI is preferred to demonstrate the presence of strategic vascular lesions because of its greater capabilities to show small lesions in regions that are difficult to image with CT, such as the globus pallidus, thalamus, and substantia nigra, and also because of the possibility to scan in different directions (eg, coronal and sagittal). The different T1- and T2-weighted sequences have their own qualities, and when combined, they give complimentary information on the characteristics and probable cause of ischemic pathology. This may be important to fulfill the diagnostic criteria mentioned earlier. T1-weighted images reveal lacunes and frontal cortical infarcts. Fluid attenuated inversion recovery (FLAIR) is best suited for the assessment of white matter lesions. It has the advantage of suppressing cerebrospinal fluid signal, allowing a simple distinction of lacunes and perivascular spaces from ischemic white matter lesions, both of which are bright on standard T2-(T)SE weighted images.[43,44] For the assessment of ischemic lesions in the thalamus and infratentorial regions, conventional T2-weighted images are preferred.[45] In addition, T2*-weighted gradient echo sequences are more sensitive for the detection of hemorrhagic lacunae than spin echo and FLAIR sequences.[46–49] An imaging protocol using T1, T2, T2*, and FLAIR images may therefore optimize diagnostic capabilities of MRI for VP (Table 1). Fig. 1 and 2 show MRI scans in patients with VP with an insidious and an acute onset.

Because subcortical lesions in the basal ganglia and the white matter can also occur in older

Table 1			
Example of imaging protocol for the detection of cerebral vascular lesions			
Coronal 3D T1 gradient echo		TR	15 ms
		TE	7 ms
		T1	500 ms
		Slice thickness	1 mm
		Flip angle	15°–30°
Axial T2 spin echo		TR	4000 ms
		TE	100 ms
		Slice thickness	3–5 mm
Axial or coronal FLAIR		TR	8000 ms
		TE	102 ms
		T1	2000 ms
		Slice thickness	3–5 mm
Axial T2* gradient echo		TR	650 ms
		TE	15 ms
		Slice thickness	3–5 mm
		Flip angle	≥20°

Abbreviations: T1, inversion time; TE, echo time; TR, repetition time.

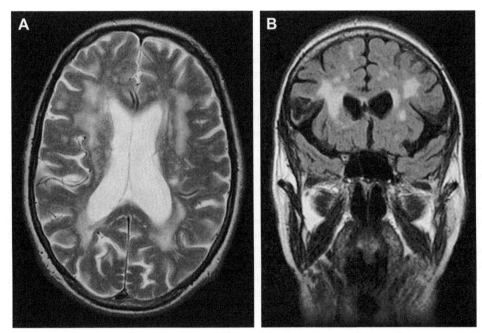

Fig. 1. Axial T2-weighted spin echo (*A*) and coronal FLAIR (*B*) MRI scan of a 67-year-old patient with VPi with a slowly, progressive frontal gait disorder showing vascular lesions diffusely in the white matter.

people without parkinsonism,[50,51] one has to relate not only the severity but also the location of lesions with clinical features. Partially or widely confluent subcortical lesions have been reported in 10% to 30% of asymptomatic elderly patients having vascular risk factors.[51,52] Vascular lesion load may serve as a marker of disease severity. Different methods can be used for the

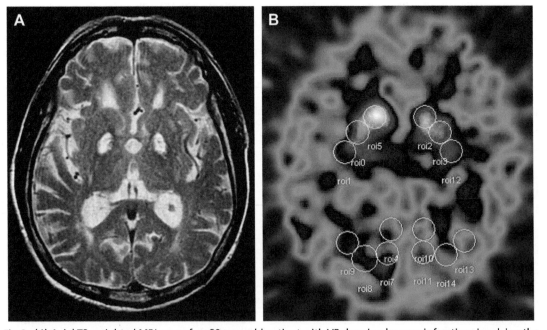

Fig. 2. (*A*) Axial T2-weighted MRI scan of an 80-year-old patient with VP showing lacunar infarctions involving the globus pallidus on both sides. Two years earlier, the patient noticed a shuffling gait and bradykinesia on both sides immediately after resuscitation. (*B*) DAT SPECT of the patient showing striatal FP-CIT uptake reduction in a similar distribution as in PD, only less asymmetrical.

measurement of ischemic white matter lesions, ranging from visual rating to fully computerized techniques. Visual rating of ischemic white matter lesions is quick, and several scales are available with good reproducibility.[53] However, the visual scales often do not provide information about size and location and are usually not linear. Furthermore, scores from different visual rating scales are not directly comparable.[54] They display ceiling effects and poor discrimination of absolute volumes. Consequently, they may be less sensitive than volumetric studies in differentiating clinical groups.[55] Volumetric studies mainly use semiautomated methods that may provide detailed information on location and size, but they are time consuming.[56] Further work is needed to make automated lesion counting more easy. The differential diagnosis of multifocal or diffuse cerebral demyelinization in adults is shown in **Box 2**.

Dopamine Transporter Single-photon Emission Computed Tomography Scan

A series of cocaine analogs have been developed successfully for imaging dopamine transporters (DATs) (eg, [^{123}I] β-CIT, [^{123}I]-FP-CIT, and

---

Box 2
Causes of multifocal or diffuse cerebral demyelinization in adults, besides small vessel disease.

Alzheimer disease

Multiple sclerosis

Progressive multifocal leukoencephalopathy

Human immunodeficiency virus encephalopathy

Creutzfeldt-Jakob disease

Hyperperfusion syndrome

Posttransfusion syndrome

Proximal myotonic myopathy

Trauma

Radiotherapy

Chemotherapy

Postinfectious demyelinization

Posthypoxic ischemic encephalopathy

Cyclosporin or other immunosuppressants

Vitamin B$_{12}$ deficiency

α-Galactosidase deficiency (Fabry disease)

Data from Van Gijn J. Leukoaraiosis and vascular dementia. Neurology 1998;51(Suppl 3):S3–8.

[99m-Tc] TRODAT) and are therefore useful in showing a reduction of presynaptic tracer uptake, which correlates with disease duration and severity of PD.[57]

A significant presynaptic dopaminergic deficit can be found in VPi and VPa groups when compared with normal controls.[21,58–63] The dopaminergic deficit in patients with VP that was demonstrated by [^{123}I] FP-CIT SPECT (single-photon emission computed tomography) is as marked as in PD, and it also affects the striatum in a pattern similar to that described in PD,[58] in which (in accordance with neuropathologic evidence of selective degeneration of nigrostriatal neurons)[64] a predominant reduction of tracer uptake is typically seen in the posterior putamen.[65] In patients with VP, the dopaminergic deficit is reflected in the caudate/putamen radioactivity ratios, similar to the PD group, which were significantly higher than in normal controls. Patients with VPi, show a presynaptic dopaminergic deficit similar to patients with VPa. Normal presynaptic tracer binding may also be found in patients with VP,[66–68] showing that VP is heterogeneous in its etiology. See **Fig. 2B** for DAT SPECT in VP.

To distinguish VP from PD, the presence of a symmetric FP-CIT uptake in the basal ganglia may help.[58] Asymmetry of degeneration of nigrostriatal dopaminergic projections to the motor striatum is a hallmark of PD that underlies the common initial asymmetry of clinical features at presentation. The mean asymmetry index that compares right to left striatal FP-CIT binding in most patients with VP, however, is normal and lower than in PD.[58] This is consistent with the idea that the disease in the vascular group usually is more diffusely distributed than in PD, and the parkinsonism is relatively symmetric in most of the patients.[10] The presence of MRI evidence of diffuse small vessel disease, in most patients, may explain this observation. Only occasionally the clinical presentation of VP at onset may be asymmetrical, especially when the disease onset is acute and SPECT is performed in the acute phase. Substantial asymmetry of presynaptic uptake reduction in patients with VP may therefore be a less common finding.[21,59–63]

Some patients with VPa may show a "punched out" FP-CIT uptake in the putamen or globus pallidus, corresponding to a focal infarction.[58,61–63]

SUMMARY

Criteria for the clinical diagnosis of VP have been proposed, which are derived from a postmortem examination study. CT and MRI can support this clinical diagnosis with positive imaging findings. One has to consider the 2 different types of onset with their related locations of lesions: an insidious onset type presenting itself with white matter lesions diffusely located in the watershed areas and an acute onset type with lesions located in contralateral strategic areas. DAT SPECT may also be of help to distinguish VP from PD and other parkinsonisms.

ACKNOWLEDGMENTS

I would like to thank Dr Th. De Jong, radiologist, of my hospital for advising me.

REFERENCES

1. Critchley M. Arteriosclerotic parkinsonism. Brain 1929;52:23–83.
2. Tolosa ES, Santamaria J. Parkinsonism and basal ganglia infarcts. Neurology 1984;34:1516–8.
3. Friedman A, Kang UJ, Tatemichi TK, et al. A case of parkinsonism following striatal lacunar infarction. J Neurol Neurosurg Psychiatr 1986;49:1087–8.
4. Thompson PD, Marsden CD. Gait disorder of subcortical arteriosclerotic encephalopathy: Binswanger's disease. Mov Disord 1987;2:1–8.
5. FitzGerald PM, Jankovic J. Lower body parkinsonism: evidence for vascular etiology. Mov Disord 1989;4:249–60.
6. Zijlmans JC, Thijssen HO, Vogels OJ, et al. MRI in patients suspected of vascular parkinsonism. Neurology 1995;45:2183–8.
7. de Rijk M, Tzourio C, Breteler M, et al. Prevalence of parkinsonism and Parkinson's disease in Europe: the EURPARKINSON collaborative study. J Neurol Neurosurg Psychiatr 1997;62:10–5.
8. Winikates J, Jankovic J. Clinical correlates of vascular parkinsonism. Arch Neurol 1999;56: 98–102.
9. Zijlmans JC, Poels PJ, Duysens J, et al. Quantitative gait analysis in patients with vascular parkinsonism. Mov Disord 1996;11(5):501–8.
10. Zijlmans J, Daniel S, Hughes A, et al. A clinico-pathological investigation of vascular parkinsonism (VP). Including clinical criteria for the diagnosis of VP. Mov Disord 2004;19:630–40.
11. DeLong MR, Wichmann T. Circuits and circuit disorders of the basal ganglia. Arch Neurol 2007;64(1): 20–4.
12. Chang CM, Yu YL, Leung SY, et al. Vascular pseudo-parkinsonism. Acta Neurol Scand 1992;86:588–92.
13. Mayo J, Arias M, Leno C, et al. Vascular parkinsonism and periarteritis nodosa. Neurology 1986; 36:874–5.
14. Tison F, Duché B, Loiseau P. Syndrome hemiparkinsonien vasculaire. [Vascular hemiparkinson syndrome]. Rev Neurol (Paris) 1993;149:565–7 [in French].
15. Lee MS, Lee SA, Heo JH, et al. A patient with a resting tremor and a lacunar infarction at the border between the thalamus and the internal capsule. Mov Disord 1993;8:244–6.
16. De La Fuente Fernandez R, Lopez J, Rey del Corral P, et al. Peduncular hallucinosis and right hemiparkinsonism caused by left mesencephalic infarction. J Neurol Neurosurg Psychiatr 1994;57: 870.
17. Pullicino P, Lichter D, Benedict R. Micrographia with cognitive dysfunction: "minimal" sequelae of a putaminal infarct. Mov Disord 1994;9:371–3.
18. Kulisevsky J, Avila A. Bipolar affective disorder and unilateral parkinsonism after a brainstem infarction. Mov Disord 1995;10:799–801.
19. Mark MH, Sage JI, Walters AS, et al. Binswanger's disease presenting as levodopa-responsive parkinsonism: clinicopathological study of three cases. Mov Disord 1995;10:450–4.
20. Reider-Grosswasser I, Bornstein N, Korczyn A. Parkinsonism in patients with lacunar infarcts of the basal ganglia. Eur Neurol 1995;35:46–9.
21. Boecker H, Weindl A, Leenders K, et al. Secondary parkinsonism due to focal substantia nigra lesions: a PET study with [^{18}F] FDG and [^{18}F] fluorodopa. Acta Neurol Scand 1996;93:387–92.
22. Fénelon G, Houéto J. Unilateral parkinsonism following a large infarct in the territory of the lenticulostriate arteries. Mov Disord 1997;12:1086–90.
23. Leduc V, Montagne B, Destée A. Parkinsonism consecutive to an hemorrhagic lesion of the substantia nigra. Mov Disord 1997;12(Suppl 1):2.
24. Alarcón F, Zijlmans JCM, Dueñas G, et al. Post-stroke movement disorders: report of 56 patients. J Neurol Neurosurg Psychiatr 2004;75:1568–74.
25. Alzheimer A. Die Seelenstörung auf arteriosclerotischer Grundlage. [Psychiatric disturbance with arteriosclerotic basis]. Z Psychiat 1902;59:695–711 [in German].
26. Blass JP, Hoher S, Nitsch R. A translation of Otto Binswanger's article, 'the delineation of the generalized progressive paralyses'. Arch Neurol 1991;48: 961–72.
27. Breteler MM, van Amerongen NM, van Swieten JC, et al. Cognitive correlates of ventricular enlargement and cerebral white matter lesions on magnetic resonance imaging. The Rotterdam study. Stroke 1994; 25:1109–15.
28. Schneider R, Ringelstein EB, Zeumer H, et al. The role of plasma hyperviscosity in subcortical arteriosclerotic encephalopathy (Binswanger's disease). J Neurol 1987;234:67–73.
29. Caplan LR, Schoene WC. Clinical features of subcortical arteriosclerotic encephalopathy (Binswanger's disease). Neurology 1978;28:1206–15.

30. Thomas D, du Boulay G, Marshall J, et al. Effect of hematocrit on cerebral blood flow in man. Lancet 1977;2:941–3.

31. Ma K, Lundberg P, Lilja A, et al. Binswanger's disease in the absence of chronic arterial hypertension: a case report with clinical, radiological and immunohistochemical observations on intracerebral blood vessels. Acta Neuropathol 1992;83:434–9.

32. van Swieten JC, Geyskes GG, Derix MM, et al. Hypertension in the elderly is associated with white matter lesions and cognitive decline. Ann Neurol 1991;30:825–30.

33. Van Gijn J. Leukoaraiosis and vascular dementia. Neurology 1998;51(Suppl 3):S3–8.

34. Rao SM, Mittenberg W, Bernardin L, et al. Neuropsychological test findings in subjects with leukoaraiosis. Arch Neurol 1989;46:40–4.

35. Boone KB, Miller BL, Lesser IM, et al. Neuropsychological correlates of white matter lesions in healthy elderly subjects. Arch Neurol 1992;49:549–54.

36. Jankovic J. Clinical aspects of Parkinson's disease. In: Marsden CD, Fahn S, editors. The assessment and therapy of parkinsonism (New trends in clinical neurology series). New Jersey (NJ): Parthenon Publishing Group; 1990. p. 53–75.

37. Hughes AJ, Daniel SE, Kilford L, et al. Accuracy of clinical diagnosis of idiopathic Parkinson's disease: a clinico-pathological study of 100 cases. J Neurol Neurosurg Psychiatr 1992;55:181–4.

38. Gilman S, Low P, Quinn N, et al. Consensus statement on the diagnosis of multiple system atrophy. J Neurol Sci 1999;163:94–8.

39. Litvan I, Agid Y, Calne D, et al. Clinical research criteria for the diagnosis of progressive supranuclear palsy (Steele-Richardson-Olszewski syndrome): report of the NINDS-SPSP International Workshop. Neurology 1996;47:1–9.

40. McKeith IG, Galasko D, Kosaka K, et al. Consensus guidelines for the clinical and pathologic diagnosis of dementia with Lewy bodies (DLB): report of the consortium on DLB international workshop. Neurology 1996 Nov;47(5):1113–24 [review].

41. Dubinsky RM, Jankovic J. Progressive supranuclear palsy and a multi-infarct state. Neurology 1987;37:570–6.

42. Winikates J, Jankovic J. Vascular progressive supranuclear palsy. J Neural Transm Suppl 1994;42:189–201.

43. Haynal JV, Bryant DJ, Kasuboski L, et al. Use of fluid attenuated inversion recovery (FLAIR) pulse sequences in MRI of the brain. J Comput Assist Tomogr 1992;16(6):841–4.

44. De Coene B, Haynal JV, Gatehouse P, et al. MR of the brain using fluid-attenuated inversion recovery (FLAIR) pulse sequences. AJNR Am J Neuroradiol 1992;13(6):1555–64.

45. Bastos Leite AJ, van Straaten EC, Scheltens P, et al. Thalamic lesions in vascular dementia: low sensitivity of fluid-attenuated inversion recovery (FLAIR) imaging. Stroke 2004;35(2):415–9.

46. Challa VR, Moody DM. The value of magnetic resonance imaging in the detection of type II hemorrhagic lacunes. Stroke 1989;20(6):822–5.

47. Fazekas F, Kleinert R, Roob G, et al. Histopathologic analysis of foci of signal loss on gradient-echo T2*-weighted MR images in patients with spontaneous intracerebral hemorrhage: evidence of microangiopathy-related microbleeds. AJNR Am J Neuroradiol 1999;20(4):637–42.

48. Kim DE, Bae HJ, Kim H, et al. Gradient echo magnetic resonance imaging in the prediction of hemorrhagic vs ischemic stroke: a need for the consideration of the extent of leukoariosis. Arch Neurol 2002;59(3):425–9.

49. Ripoll MA, Sjösteen B, Hartman M, et al. MR detectability and appearance of small experimental intracranial hematomas at 1.5 T and 0.5 T. A 6-7-month follow-up study. Acta Radiol 2003;44(2):199–205.

50. Fisher CM. Lacunes: small, deep cerebral infarcts. Neurology 1965;15:774–84.

51. Awad IA, Spetzler RF, Hodak JA, et al. Incidental subcortical lesions identified on magnetic resonance imaging in the elderly. 1. Correlation with age and cerebrovascular risk factors. Stroke 1986;17:1084–9.

52. Fazekas F. Magnetic resonance signal abnormalities in asymptomatic individuals: their incidence and functional correlates. Eur Neurol 1989;29:164–8.

53. Scheltens P, Erkinjunti T, Leys D, et al. White matter changes on CT and MRI: an overview of visual rating scales. European Task Force on Age-Related White Matter Changes. Eur Neurol 1998;39(2):80–9.

54. Pantoni L, Simoni M, Pracucci G, et al. Visual rating scales for age-related white matter changes (leukoaraiosis): can the heterogeneity be reduced? Stroke 2002;33(12):2827–33.

55. van Straaten EC, Fazekas F, Rostrup E, et al. Impact of white matter hyperintensities scoring method on correlations with clinical data: the LADIS study. Stroke 2006;37(3):836–40.

56. Anbeek P, Vincken KL, van Bochove GS, et al. Probabilistic segmentation of brain tissue in MR imaging. Neuroimage 2005;27(4):795–804.

57. Booij J, Tissingh G, Winogrodzka A, et al. Imaging of the dopaminergic neurotransmission system using single-photon emission tomography and positron emission tomography in patients with parkinsonism. Eur J Nucl Med 1999;26(2):171–82.

58. Zijlmans J, Evans A, Fontes F, et al. [123I] FP-CIT SPECT study of vascular parkinsonism and Parkinson's disease. Mov Disord 2007;22(9):1278–85.

59. Peters S, Eising EG, Przuntek H, et al. Vascular parkinsonism: a case report and review of the literature. J Clin Neurosci 2001;8(3):268–71.

60. Remy P, de Recondo A, Defer G, et al. Peduncular 'rubral' tremor and dopaminergic denervation: a PET study. Neurology 1995;45:472–7.

61. Marshall V, Grosset D. Role of dopamine transporter imaging in routine clinical practice. Mov Disord 2003;18(12):1415–23.

62. Peralta C, Werner P, Holl B, et al. Parkinsonism following striatal infarcts: incidence in a prospective stroke unit cohort. J Neural Transm 2004;111:1473–83.

63. Plotkin M, Amthauer H, Quill S, et al. Imaging of dopamine transporters and D2 receptors in vascular parkinsonism: a report of four cases. J Neural Transm 2005;112:1355–61.

64. Fearnley JM, Lees AJ. Aging and Parkinson's disease: substantia nigra regional selectivity. Brain 1991;114:2283–301.

65. Loberboym M, Djaldetti R, Melamed E, et al. 123I-FP-CIT SPECT imaging of dopamine transporters in patients with cerebrovascular disease and clinical diagnosis of vascular parkinsonism. J Nucl Med 2004;45(10):1688–93.

66. Brooks DJ, Ibanez V, Sawle GV, et al. Differing patterns of striatal 18F-dopa uptake in Parkinson's disease, multiple system atrophy, and progressive supranuclear palsy. Ann Neurol 1990;28(4):547–55.

67. Tzen KY, Lu CS, Yen TC, et al. Differential diagnosis of Parkinson's disease and vascular parkinsonism by (99m)Tc-TRODAT-1. J Nucl Med 2001;42(3):408–13.

68. Gerschlager W, Bencsits G, Pirker W, et al. [123I]beta-CIT SPECT distinguishes vascular parkinsonism from Parkinson's disease. Mov Disord 2002;17(3):518–23.

Role of Neuroimaging in the Evaluation of Tremor

Davina J. Hensman, MA, MBBS, Peter G. Bain, MA, MBBS, MD, FRCP*

KEYWORDS

- Essential tremor • Dystonic tremor • Holmes tremor
- Orthostatic tremor • Deep brain stimulation

Standard magnetic resonance (MR) and CT imaging has had a limited role in the routine management of tremulous patients except mainly for people with Holmes tremor syndrome and other secondary causes of tremor (multiple sclerosis or Wilson disease).

The new millennium has seen the introduction of single photon emission CT (SPECT) imaging techniques, particularly ^{123}I-FP-CIT (iodine 123-labelled N-ω-fluoropropyl-2β-carbomethoxy-3β-[4-iodophenyl]nortropane) SPECT (DaTSCAN), into routine clinical practice as a means of assessing the integrity of the nigrostriatal dopaminergic system in patients with tremor. Care is required in the analysis of DaTSCAN scans, which can be reported visually; semiquantitatively, using a region of interest approach; or quantitatively, using statistical parametric mapping. Furthermore, caution should be exercised when interpreting an abnormal DaTSCAN result and scan findings should be compared to clinical signs to determine whether or not they are congruous.[1]

The introduction of first ^{18}F-dopa ([fluorine-18] fluorodopa) positron emission tomography (PET) and then DaTSCAN scanning into clinical trial work has even led to a new class of "parkinsonian" patient termed a subject with a *scan without evidence of dopaminergic deficits* (SWEDDs). These patients have subsequently been carefully assessed and preliminary information indicates that many of these SWEDDs patients have underlying dystonic tremor syndromes, an area of considerable clinical interest.

ESSENTIAL TREMOR

Classical essential tremor consists of a bilateral, visible, persistent, and largely symmetrical postural and/or kinetic tremor involving the hands and forearms. Essential tremor should not be diagnosed in the presence of other abnormal signs, except for subtle cognitive deficits and mildly impaired tandem gait, which have been documented in some cases.[2,3] Routine CT and MR imaging of patients with essential tremor have not shown any consistent abnormalities, whilst voxel-based morphometry revealed adaptive changes in brain structure but no signs of cerebellar degeneration in essential tremor.[4] In addition, diffusion-weighted imaging of patients with essential tremor found no differences in any of the regions of interest compared with healthy control subjects.[5] DaTSCAN studies demonstrate similar results in essential tremor to those for healthy control subjects, making it possible to distinguish essential tremor from Parkinson disease, as tracer uptake into the putamen and caudate is abnormal in the latter.[6,7] In a phase III multicenter study of DaTSCAN involving 158 patients with a clinical diagnosis of parkinsonism, 27 with essential tremor, and 35 healthy volunteers, the sensitivity for parkinsonism was 95% and specificity for essential tremor 93% (based on a consensus blinded read by a five-person panel).[7] Thus current experience indicates that DaTSCAN is a valuable tool in the differentiation of essential tremor from Parkinson disease (Fig. 1).

Work related to this article was supported with funding from the National Tremor Foundation, Rosetree's Trust, Muirhead Trust, and the Hammersmith Hospitals Special Trustees (all United Kingdom charities).
Department of Neurosciences, Charing Cross Hospital, London W6 8RP, UK
* Corresponding author.
E-mail address: p.bain@ic.ac.uk (P.G. Bain).

Neuroimag Clin N Am 20 (2010) 77–86
doi:10.1016/j.nic.2009.08.005

neuroimaging.theclinics.com

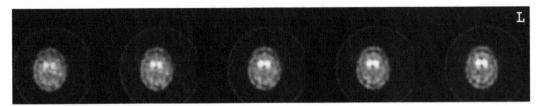

Fig. 1. DaTSCAN image from a patient with parkinsonism demonstrating reduced bilateral putaminal tracer uptake. Good caudate uptake remains, giving the impression of two "periods." In a normal DaTSCAN, the appearance should resemble two "commas".

PET and functional MR imaging studies have demonstrated bilateral activation in the cerebellum, red nucleus, and thalamus of patients with essential tremor, meanwhile, two ^{1}H-MRS (proton MR spectroscopy) studies have indicated that there is a selective reduction of the neuronal marker N-acetyl-aspartate in the cerebellum of essential tremor patients, in keeping with a converging view that a disturbance of the corticocerebellothalmocortical loop is the pathophysiological mechanism underlying essential tremor.[4,8–11]

Using ^{123}I-metaiodobenzylguanidine (MIBG) cardiac scintigraphy, abnormalities have been recently detected in patients with Parkinson disease.[12] However, this technique revealed no abnormalities in essential tremor patients.[13]

A difficult clinical scenario involves patients with long-standing essential tremor (decades) who then develop features of parkinsonism. The issue then arises as to whether mild parkinsonian features are manifestations of long-standing essential tremor, superimposed age-related changes, or Parkinson disease that has developed on top of essential tremor. Hensman and colleagues (2006)[14] evaluated the role of DaTS-CAN imaging in 20 patients with essential tremor and features of parkinsonism and found that 50% had abnormal scans (Fig. 2). The clinical features of these patients were similar to those with normal DaTSCANs except that they had rest-tremor magnitudes that exceeded that of their intention tremors or had bradykinesia, rest tremor, and rigidity.

ISOLATED REST TREMORS AND LONG-DURATION ASYMMETRIC POSTURAL TREMORS

Patients with isolated unilateral tremor, without other features of parkinsonism, provide a difficult diagnostic problem. These patients could have a dystonic tremor syndrome; a highly atypical variant of essential tremor, which is classically symmetric; or benign tremulous Parkinson disease. A ^{18}F-dopa PET study involving 8 patients with hereditary essential tremor, 12 with sporadic essential tremor, and 11 with predominantly rest tremor demonstrated normal tracer uptake into the putamen in all the hereditary and 10 of the 12 sporadic essential tremor cases. However, in all the patients with rest tremor, there was a marked reduction of the ^{18}F-dopa influx constant (Ki) to levels associated with Parkinson disease.[15]

A long-term study of 13 patients originally presenting with an asymmetric postural tremor (diagnosed as "essential tremor" with or without mild rest tremor) revealed that these patients subsequently developed Parkinson disease. The clinical findings were supported in 5 of the 13 patients using β-CIT (Iodine 123 labelled 2β-carboxymethyl-3β-[4-iodophenyl]tropane) SPECT, indicating that at least some cases of "essential tremor" do develop Parkinson disease.[16] However, the study was subject to bias because the development of Parkinson disease was an entry criterion for the study.[17] More recently, a study clarified this issue showing that about 50% of essential tremor patients who developed features of parkinsonism

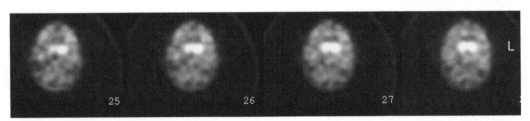

Fig. 2. Axial DaTSCAN images showing reduced uptake in the putamina bilaterally from a patient with long-standing essential tremor who subsequently developed features of parkinsonism, indicating the development of Parkinson disease on top of essential tremor.

have abnormal DaTSCAN scans, suggesting that either they have had underlying Parkinson disease or have developed Parkinson disease. However, 40% had normal DaTSCAN imaging and in 20% the scan was equivocal.[14]

DYSTONIC TREMOR SYNDROMES

Tremor is often apparent in patients with primary or secondary dystonia. It is termed *dystonic tremor* if the tremor occurs in a body part also affected by dystonia and *tremor associated with dystonia* when tremor occurs in a body part not affected by dystonia but dystonia is present elsewhere.[18] These two types of tremor commonly coexist in patients with a dystonic tremor syndrome.[19]

In the primary dystonic tremor syndromes, routine cerebral MR and CT imaging are usually normal. Although dystonic tremor and tremor associated with dystonia are typically action tremors, with a tendency to enhance during attempts to perform fine manual tasks, these conditions can cause a rest tremor and a clinical picture that resembles Parkinson disease.[20] Some patients with a dystonic tremor have parkinsonian signs that include hypomimia, reduced arm swing, asymmetric rest and postural tremor, increased limb tone, and abnormally slow and small repetitive finger movements.[21] Consequently, differentiation of patients with dystonic tremor syndromes from those with Parkinson disease becomes an important clinical issue. Perhaps this is where DaTSCAN imaging can be particularly helpful, as it is abnormal in Parkinson disease and reported normal in the dystonic tremor syndromes.[19–21]

Dystonic tremor may be associated with an underlying condition (eg, Wilson disease [see below]) or, rarely, a structural cerebral lesion, as in the case of a focal parietal lesion (posttraumatic cerebromalacia) reported to result in dystonic head tremor and an anterior thalamic infarct contralateral dystonic hand tremor.[22,23]

SUBJECTS WITH SCANS WITHOUT EVIDENCE OF DOPAMINERGIC DEFICITS

Four to fifteen percent of patients entered into several randomized trials of dopaminergic medication for Parkinson disease were found to have normal presynaptic nigrostriatal dopaminergic imaging and were termed *SWEDDs*. These patients had several features of parkinsonism that had lead neurologists to not only diagnose but to enter these patients into randomized controlled trials involving medical treatments for Parkinson disease. However, dopaminergic

imaging of these patients, up to 4 years later, was normal and withdrawal of levodopa had no deleterious effect on their clinical state.[24–26] Consequently, this has led to considerable interest about the nature of the condition or conditions underlying these SWEDDs patients.

Recently, data has emerged that at least some of these SWEDDs patients have dystonic tremor and that this had been misdiagnosed as Parkinson disease.[19–21] However, whether this proves to be the case for the majority of SWEDDs patients remains to be seen.

PRIMARY ORTHOSTATIC TREMOR

Primary orthostatic tremor is a high-frequency tremor that predominantly involves the legs and trunk whilst in the standing position.[27,28] Electrophysiology plays a major role in the diagnosis of orthostatic tremor as it has a characteristic frequency (13–18 Hz).[29] Four modalities of imaging have been used to investigate orthostatic tremor: PET, SPECT, MR imaging, and transcranial sonography. The interpretation of both sonography and functional imaging depends on whether primary orthostatic tremor is thought to be associated with dopaminergic deficit: a controversial topic.[30]

In a study of four patients with primary orthostatic tremor in which PET was coregistered with MR imaging, bilateral cerebellar hemisphere activation and significant activation of the cerebellar vermis, left lentiform nucleus, and left thalamus were detected. The investigators postulated that cerebellar activation is a feature common to all tremors, and that tremors may be associated with overactivity of a common circuit involving cerebellothalamic connections.[31]

Functional imaging of the nigrostriatal dopaminergic pathway using DaTSCAN has in some studies suggested that orthostatic tremor was associated with a dopaminergic deficit and hence changes on SPECT.[32] However, recent reports indicate that this is not always the case.[33,34] Katzenschlager and colleagues[32] detected a dopaminergic deficit in orthostatic tremor. This was more evenly distributed than in Parkinson disease and affected all parts of the striatum nearly evenly. They found that, unlike in Parkinson disease, there was no correlation between the extent or distribution of tracer uptake and disease duration or severity. However, it is possible that there was some suppression of tracer uptake, as these patients were on co-beneldopa prior to investigation. Nevertheless, the investigators suggest that a presynaptic dopaminergic deficit is unlikely to be the primary underlying cause of the pathophysiology of orthostatic tremor and speculate that a central primary generator causes orthostatic tremor and a modulation of the dopaminergic system. In this regard, Trocello and colleagues[33] found no significant difference between the controls and patients with orthostatic tremor and postulate that there are different subtypes of orthostatic tremor:

Type A—without dopaminergic loss
Type B—with mild dopaminergic loss without parkinsonian symptoms
Type C—orthostatic tremor associated with Parkinson disease

The concept of a disease spectrum in orthostatic tremor is supported by the variable response of patients to levodopa.[35]

No MR image changes characteristic of orthostatic tremor have been described. In a study of the clinical and neurophysiologic findings in 26 subjects with orthostatic tremor, 13 patients had MR imaging scans.[36] Of these 13 cases, the MR image scans were normal in 9, showed microvascular ischemic disease in 2, an old infarct in the right posterior temporoparietal lobe in 1, and mild diffuse atrophy in 1.

A transcranial sonographic study of four orthostatic tremor patients found hyperechogenic substantia nigra, a finding that also occurs in Parkinson disease.[37]

NEUROPATHIC TREMOR

Neuropathic tremor is most commonly seen in patients with demyelinating peripheral neuropathies. It is usually a postural or kinetic tremor affecting distal rather than proximal muscles. It is most frequently seen in patients with IgM demyelinating paraproteinaemic neuropathy. These patients had normal cerebral MR imaging and most had normal central motor conduction times assessed with magnetic brain stimulation.[38]

Detailed neurophysiological studies of patients with IgM demyelinating paraproteinaemic neuropathy have suggested that tremor arises because a central processor is misled by distorted mistimed peripheral inputs into producing tremor.[38] PET activation studies have shown that the cerebellar hemispheres are hyperactive bilaterally, both during tremor and at rest, in these patients.[39] There are no other reports of detectable abnormalities on neuroimaging of patients with neuropathic tremor.

DRUG-INDUCED TREMORS

Tremors occur in the context of drug-induced parkinsonism (DIP), which may result from centrally acting antiemetics and antipsychotics.[40] Differentiating DIP from Parkinson disease can be difficult, particularly as clinical descriptions of DIP differ.[41,42] Postsynaptic imaging shows D2 receptor blockade and it was expected that presynaptic imaging would be normal, as found in three DIP patients.[43–45] However, in one DaTS-CAN study, 5 of 7 patients with a differential diagnosis of DIP versus Parkinson disease had abnormal scans. In another report, 11 of 20 patients with DIP had abnormal scans, which were characterized by diminished binding in the caudate and putamen.[34,42] Reversibility of parkinsonism after neuroleptic withdrawal is variable and three clinical scenarios have been proposed:

DIP with no relationship to Parkinson disease
DIP that unmasks Parkinson disease
DIP that antedates Parkinson disease

The latter two scenarios may account for the dopaminergic deficits described.[34,40,42]

HOLMES TREMOR SYNDROME

Holmes tremor syndrome has in the past been labeled *rubral tremor*, *midbrain tremor*, *thalamic tremor*, *myorythmia*, and *Benedikt syndrome*. It is named after Gordon Holmes, who first gave an accurate description of the characteristics of this type of tremor.[46] It may arise from various underlying structural disorders, including stroke, vascular malformations, tumors, nonketotic hyperglycemia, and infections (eg, herpes simplex type 1 cerebral pedunculitis or a toxoplasma abscess in the context of HIV).[18] It is rarely present in multiple sclerosis, which tends to induce an action tremor.[47] In Holmes tremor syndromes, the lesions are most usually sited in the midbrain (Fig. 3), although lesions in the thalamus have also been described. There is a variable delay (typically 2 weeks to 2 years) between that lesion and the first appearance of Holmes tremor, which often involves proximal and distal upper limb muscles and consists of an irregular low-frequency (<4.5 Hz) rest and intention tremor and, in many cases, a postural tremor.[2,18] DaTSCAN and ^{18}F-dopa PET studies have demonstrated reduced tracer uptake in the ipsilateral putamen and caudate nuclei (Fig. 4), and current evidence suggests that, in most cases, Holmes tremor arises from lesions that interrupt the dentate-thalamic and also the nigrostriatal tracts, thus causing both an action and a rest tremor.[2,18,34]

WILSON DISEASE

Wilson disease is an autosomal recessive disease of copper metabolism resulting in the accumulation

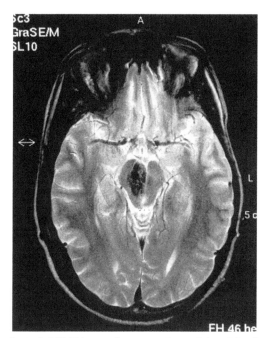

Fig. 3. Axial MR image demonstrating a right midbrain ependymoma, treated with radiotherapy, in a patient with levodopa-responsive Holmes tremor affecting the left arm.

of copper in many organs and tissues.[48] It has primarily hepatic and neurological manifestations, which include dystonia, tremor, apraxia, ataxia, dysarthria, and dysphagia.[48,49] The commonest CT scan abnormalities in Wilson disease are ventricular dilatation, cortical atrophy and brain stem atrophy or hypodensity.[49–51] CT is less sensitive than MR imaging at detecting grey and white matter changes in Wilson disease.[52]

Diverse changes on MR imaging have been reported (Table 1). The majority of studies demonstrate that abnormal findings are predominantly present in Wilson disease patients with neurological or psychiatric symptoms.[53–56] However, midbrain atrophy was found in both hepatic and neurological Wilson disease cases.[57] In a report of 12 patients, 6 of whom had mainly postural tremor, a significant correlation between Unified Parkinson Disease Rating Scale Part III (UPDRS-III) action tremor score and T2/T2*-weighted lesions of globus pallidus, substantia nigra, and head of the caudate nucleus was found in symptomatic Wilson disease patients, suggesting that basal ganglia lesions play a critical role in Wilson disease action tremor generation.[58] By contrast, a study of 47 Wilson disease patients showed that those with tremors, ataxia, dysarthria, and reduced functional capacity had thalamic lesions; whilst another report found no relationship between extrapyramidal tract involvement and neurologic type of Wilson disease (pseudoparkinsonian, dystonic, cerebellar, or asymptomatic).[52,59] Some of the variability between studies may be attributed to variability in lengths of treatment, and whether patients with hepatic Wilson disease were included or excluded. MR imaging has been used in conjunction with electromyography to suggest that postural tremor in Wilson disease is mediated through a pathological oscillatory drive from the primary motor cortex.[58]

Nigrostriatal dopaminergic dysfunction detectable with ^{18}F-dopa PET is a feature of Wilson disease and is mainly limited to patients with neurological manifestations of the disease.[60–62] Two anatomical patterns of involvement have been demonstrated in Wilson disease using ^{18}F-fluorodeoxyglucose (FDG) PET: (1) low-glucose utilization in the caput nuclei caudati and thalamic region and high consumption in the midbrain and cerebellum and (2) higher values in the caput nuclei caudati and thalamic region but lower rates in midbrain and cerebellum.[61] A case report showed some reversibility of decreased glucose metabolism on treatment.[63]

Dopaminergic deficit in Wilson disease is both pre- and postsynaptic, and is correlated with symptom severity.[64,65] SPECT appears to be

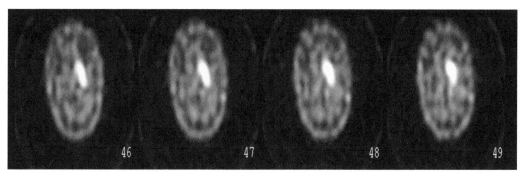

Fig. 4. Axial DaTSCAN images showing unilateral absence of tracer uptake in the putamen and caudate of a patient with Holmes tremor.

Table 1
Summary of brain areas found to have MR image changes in Wilson disease

Area	Percentage of Patients Having Change							
	Sinha et al 2006 (100 Patients)	King et al 1996 (25 Patients)	Saatci et al 1997 (30 Patients)	Roh et al 1994 (25 Patients)	Taly et al 2007 (40 Patients)	Favrole et al 2005[a] (13 Patients)	van Wassenaer-van Hall et al 1995 (49 Patients)	Das et al 2006 (15 Patients)
Cerebral atrophy	70	59	100	88	85			
Cerebellum atrophy	66	50			57.5			
Brainstem atrophy	52				70			
Basal Ganglia	86							
Putamen	72	86	85.7	68	77.5	84.6	36.7	80
Globus pallidus	40	9	88.8	20	37.5		22.4	60
Caudate	61	45	42.8		62.5		8.2	80
Thalamus	58	54	47.6	92	60	76.9	16.3	53.3
Midbrain	49	77	76.2	76	52.5			46.7
Substantia nigra		41						
Tegmentum		64						
Red nuclei		32					2.0	
Crura		4.5						
Inferior tectum		14					8.2	
Face of giant panda					10			
Pons	20	82	85.7	68	25	84.6	14.3 (base)	33.3
Cerebellum	10	50			7.5		8.2	
Mesencephalon						84.6	22.4	
Corpus callosum								
Internal capsule						92.3	14.3 (posterior limb)	
Cortex								40
Cerebral white matter	59			4	20			53.3

[a] Fluid-attenuated inversion recovery data.

more sensitive to Wilson disease–related changes than MR imaging.[53] By correlating ^{99m}Tc-ethyl-cysteinate dimer (ECD) SPECT with MR imaging, a dysfunction of frontotemporal and parietooccipital cortical areas was demonstrated, highlighting the involvement of the basal ganglia-premotor cortex and supplementary motor area circuitry in Wilson disease pathophysiology.[53]

Transcranial sonography detected lenticular nucleus and thalamic hyperechogenicity in neurologically symptomatic and asymptomatic Wilson disease patients, and findings correlated with disease severity.[66]

CEREBELLAR TREMORS

Cerebellar lesions predominantly provoke action tremors, including intention, kinetic, and postural tremors. These are often accompanied by other signs of cerebellar disease, namely nystagmus, dysarthria, dysmetria, dysdiadochokinesia, and ataxia. The most common causes of cerebellar tremor are multiple sclerosis, trauma, degenerative diseases (spinocerebellar ataxias), tumors, paraneoplastic syndromes, and toxins (eg, alcoholism, lithium, and anticonvulsants). As a general rule, toxins cause bilateral action tremors. MR imaging of the brain is recommended.[67]

In patients with fragile X tremor ataxia syndrome (FXTAS), which is caused by a 55–200 CGG repeat expansion in the fragile X mental retardation 1 gene (*FMR 1*), hyperintensity may be visible in the middle cerebellar peduncles, the "MCP" sign (Fig. 5).[68]

PSYCHOGENIC TREMOR

Seventy-five percent of patients with psychogenic tremor are female and it is the most common form of psychogenic movement disorder. The diagnosis is largely based on the clinical history and careful observations of the patient's tremor and there are various phenomena indicative of psychogenic tremor.[69] However, because parkinsonian and other organic tremors can present at times of great stress, it is prudent to assess patients with suspected psychogenic tremor using MR and dopamine transporter imaging.[2]

NEUROIMAGING OF DEEP BRAIN STIMULATION AND LESIONAL SURGERY FOR TREMOR

Thalamotomy has been widely deployed for the treatment of severe medically refractory tremulous conditions, including Parkinson disease, essential tremor, multiple sclerosis–associated tremor, dystonic tremor, Holmes tremor syndrome, and primary writing tremor. Originally, lesions were

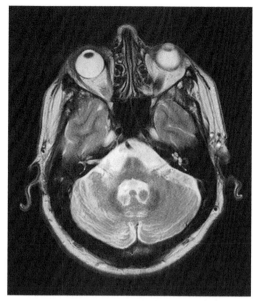

Fig. 5. T2-weighted axial MR image at the level of the internal auditory meati showing ill-defined hyperintensity in both middle cerebellar peduncles (the "MCP" sign) and loss of volume in the pons and middle cerebellar peduncles (no pathological enhancement was demonstrated).

placed stereotactically, with the aid of ventriculography, in the nucleus ventralis intermedius and/or ventralis oralis posterior. However, with the advent

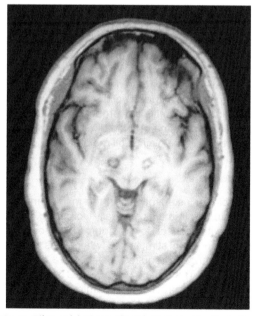

Fig. 6. Bilateral lesions placed stereotactically in the region of the subthalamic nuclei in a patient with advanced Parkinson disease.

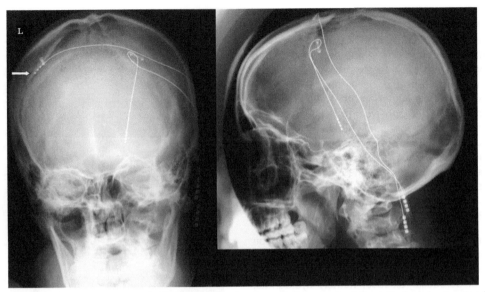

Fig. 7. Anteroposterior and lateral skull radiographs showing displacement of the left deep brain stimulation electrode from the thalamus to just under the skull (*arrow*). The right-side electrode remains correctly in situ within the thalamus.

of deep brain stimulation and MR/CT image fusion systems providing both increased accuracy and safety, the focus has moved onto the zona incerta and the subthalamic nucleus for the treatment of tremors (**Fig. 6**).[70] Furthermore, postoperative MR imaging is now routinely used prior to initiating stimulation to check that the deep brain stimulation electrodes have been accurately placed.

Occasionally, a sudden return of severe tremor and parkinsonism, if this was present preoperatively, indicates a fault in the deep brain stimulation system. This is usually the result of battery failure, accidental switching off of the stimulator by an external magnetic field, or an electrical fault in the leads or electrodes, which can be identified by interrogation of the stimulator with a physician's programmer. Rarely, the problem is caused by marked displacement of an electrode, which can be detected on a plain skull radiograph (**Fig. 7**).[70]

SUMMARY

The role for neuroimaging in the management of patients with tremor is gradually increasing, particularly with respect to stereotactic neurosurgery and deep brain stimulation, where less than 2-mm tolerance is required for accurate electrode placement. The routine use of SPECT technology to image the nigrostriatal dopaminergic system is proving helpful in the distinction of essential and dystonic tremors from neurodegenerative forms of parkinsonism and in improving our understanding of the pathophysiology of rarer tremors.

ACKNOWLEDGMENTS

We would like to thank Dr John Frank and Mr David Towey from the Department of Nuclear Medicine, Charing Cross Hospital, The National Tremor Foundation, and The Rosetree's Trust for their support and facilitation of our work.

REFERENCES

1. Hensman DJ, Frank JW, Bain PG. Systematic assessment of incongruities in the correlation between the clinical signs and DAT imaging in parkinsonism. Mov Disord 2006;21(Suppl 15):P1083.
2. Bain PG. Tremor. Parkinsonism Relat Disord 2007; 13(Suppl 3):369–74.
3. Elble RJ. Report from a US conference on essential tremor. Mov Disord 2006;21:2052–61.
4. Daniels C, Peller M, Wolff S, et al. Voxel-based morphometry shows no decreases in cerebellar gray matter volume in essential tremor. Neurology 2006;67:1452–6.
5. Martinelli P, Rizzo G, Manners D, et al. Diffusion weighted imaging study of patients with essential tremor. Mov Disord 2007;23:1182–5.
6. Booij J, Tissingh G, Boer GJ, et al. ^{123}I-FP-CIT SPECT shows pronounced decline of striatal dopamine transporter labelling in early and advanced Parkinson's disease. J Neurol Neurosurg Psychiatr 1997;62:133–40.
7. Benamer HTS, Patterson J, Grosset DG. Accurate differentiation of parkinsonism and essential tremor using visual assessmet of ^{123}I-FP-CIT SPECT

imaging: the ^{123}I-FP-CIT SPECT Study Group. Mov Disord 2000;15(3):503–10.

8. Jenkins IH, Bain PG, Colebatch JG, et al. A PET study of essential tremor: evidence for overactivity of cerebellar connections. Ann Neurol 1993;34:82–90.

9. Bucher SF, Seelos KC, Dodel RC, et al. Activation mapping in essential tremor with functional magnetic resonance imaging. Ann Neurol 1997;41:32–40.

10. Louis ED, Shungu DC, Chan S, et al. Metabolic abnormality in the cerebellum in patients with essential tremor: a proton magnetic resonance spectroscopic imaging study. Neurosci Lett 2002;333: 17–20.

11. Pagan FL, Butman JA, Dambrosia JM, et al. Evaluation of essential tremor with multi-voxel magnetic resonance spectroscopy. Neurology 2003;60: 1344–7.

12. Nagayama H, Hamamoto M, Ueda M, et al. Reliability of MIBG myocardial scintigraphy in the diagnosis of Parkinson's disease. J Neurol Neurosurg Psychiatr 2005;76:249–51.

13. Lee PH, Kim JW, Bang OY, et al. Cardiac ^{123}I-MIBG scintigraphy in patients with essential tremor. Mov Disord 2006;21:1235–8.

14. Hensman DJ, Frank JW, Towey DJ, et al. Dopamine transporter imaging of patients with essential tremor and features of parkinsonism. Mov Disord 2006; 21(Suppl 15):P1369.

15. Brooks DJ, Playford ED, Ibanez V, et al. Isolated tremor and disruption of the nigrostriatal dopaminergic system in ^{18}F-dopa PET study. Neurology 1992;42:1554–60.

16. Chaudhuri KR, Buxton-Thomas M, et al. Long duration asymmetric postural tremor is likely to predict development of Parkinson's disease and not essential tremor: clinical follow up study of 13 cases. J Neurol Neurosurg Psychiatr 2005;76:115–7.

17. Grosset DG, Lees AJ. Long duration asymmetric postural tremor in the development of Parkinson's disease. J Neurol Neurosurg Psychiatr 2005;76:9.

18. Deuschl G, Bain PG, Brin MX, an Ad Hoc Scientific Committee. Consensus statement of the movement disorder society on tremor. Mov Disord 1998;13:2–23.

19. Hawkes E, Bain PG. The clinical characteristics of dystonic tremor syndromes. Parkinsonism RelatDisord 2007;13(S2):S68 (P1.261).

20. Hensman DJ, Bain PG. Levodopa can worsen tremor associated with dystonia. Mov Disord 2006; 21:1778–80.

21. Schneider SA, Edwards MJ, Mir P, et al. Patients with adult-onset dystonic tremor resembling parkinsonian tremor have scans without evidence of dopaminergic deficit (SWEDDs). Mov Disord 2007;22: 2210–5.

22. Kim JW, Lee PH. Dystonic head tremor associated with a parietal lesion. Eur J Neurol 2007;14:e32–3.

23. Cho C, Samkoff LM. A lesion of the anterior thalamus producing dystonic hand tremor. Arch Neurol 2000; 57(9):1353–5.

24. Marek KL, Seiby J, Parkinson Study Group. B-CIT scans without evidence of dopaminergic deficit (SWEDD) in ELLDOPA-CIT and CALM-CIT study: long-term imaging. Neurology 2003;60(Suppl 1):A298.

25. Marek K, Jennings D, Seibyl J. Long term follow-up of patients with scans without evidence of dopaminergic deficit (SWEDD) in the ELLDOPA study. Neurology 2005;64(Suppl 1):A274.

26. Marshall VL, Patterson J, Hadley DM, et al. Successful antiparkinsonian medication withdrawal in patients with parkinsonism and normal FP-CIT SPECT. Mov Disord 2006;21:2247–50.

27. Heilman KM. Orthostatic tremor. Arch Neurol 1984; 41:880–1.

28. Pazzaglia P, Sabattini L, Lugaresi E. Su di un singulare disturbodeura stazione eretta (osservazione di tri casi) [On a singular disturbance of upright stance (observation of 3 cases)]. Riv Freniatr 1970; 96:450–7 [in Italian].

29. Deuschl G, Krack P, Lauk M, et al. Clinical neurophysiology of tremor. J Clin Neurophysiol 1996; 13(2):110–21.

30. Bhattacharyya KB, Basu S, Roy AD, et al. Orthostatic tremor: report of a case and review of the literature. Neurol India 2003;51:91–3.

31. Wills AJ, Thompson PD, Findley LJ, et al. A positron emission tomography study of primary orthostatic tremor. Neurology 1996;46:747–52.

32. Katzenschlager R, Costa D, Gerschlager W, et al. Dopamine transporter imaging with 123I-FP-CIT-SPECT demonstrates dopaminergic deficit in orthostatic tremor. Ann Neurol 2003;53:489–96.

33. Trocello J-M, Zanotti-Fregonasa P, Roze E, et al. Dopaminergic deficit is not the rule in orthostatic tremor. Mov Disord 2008;23:1733–8.

34. Hensman DJ, Frank JW, Bain PG. Dopamine transporter imaging of tremulous disorders. Mov Disord 2006;21(Suppl):P1367.

35. Gerschlager W, Muchau A, Katzenschlager R, et al. Natural history and syndromic associations of orthostatic tremor: a review of 41 patients. Mov Disord 2004;19:788–95.

36. Piboolnurak P, Yu QP, Pullman SL. Clinical and neurophysiologic spectrum of orthostatic tremor: case series of 26 subjects. Mov Disord 2005;20: 1455–61.

37. Spiegel J, Behnke S, Fuss G, et al. Echogenic substantia nigra in patients with orthostatic tremor. J Neural Transm 2005;112:915–20.

38. Bain PG, Britton TC, Jenkins IH, et al. Tremor associated with benign IgM paraproteinaemic neuropathy. Brain 1996;119:789–99.

39. Brooks DJ, Jenkins IH, Bain PG, et al. A comparison of the abnormal patterns of cerebral activation

associated with neuropathic and essential tremor. Neurology 1992;42(Suppl 3):423.

40. Tolosa E, Coelho M, Gallardo M. DAT imaging in drug-induced and psychogenic parkinsonism. Mov Disord 2003;18(Suppl 7):S28–33.

41. Hardie RJ, Lees AJ. Neuroleptic-induced Parkinson's syndrome: clinical features and results of treatment with levodopa. J Neurol Neurosurg Psychiatry 1988;51:850–4.

42. Lorberboym M, Treves TA, Melamed E, et al. [123I]-FP-CIT SPECT imaging for distinguishing drug-induced parkinsonism from Parkinson's disease. Mov Disord 2006;21:510–4.

43. Booij J, Speelman JD, Horstink MW, et al. The clinical benefit of imaging striatal dopamine transporters with [123I]FP-CIT SPET in differentiating patients with presynaptic parkinsonism from those with other forms of parkinsonism. Eur J Nucl Med 2001;28:266–72.

44. Kemp PM. Imaging the dopaminergic system in suspected parkinsonism, drug induced movement disorders, and Lewy body dementia. Nucl Med Commun 2005;26:87–96.

45. Scherfler C, Schwarz J, Antonini A, et al. Role of DAT-SPECT in the diagnostic work up of parkinsonism. Mov Disord 2007;22:1229–38.

46. Holmes G. On certain tremors in organic cerebral lesions. Brain 1904;27:327–75.

47. Alusi S, Glickman S, Worthington J, et al. A study of tremor in multiple sclerosis. Brain 2001;124:720–30.

48. Kitzberger R, Madl C, Ferenci P. Wilson disease. Metab Brain Dis 2005;20(4):295–302.

49. Taly AB, Meenakshi-Sundaram S, Sinha S, et al. Wilson disease description of 282 patients evaluated over 3 decades. Medicine 2007;82:112–21.

50. Williams FJB, Walsh JM. Wilson's disease and analysis of the cranial computerized tomographic appearances found in 60 patients and the changes in response with chelating agents. Brain 1981;104:735–52.

51. Jha SK, Behari M, Ahuja GK. Wilson's disease: clinical and radiological features. J Assoc Physicians India 1998;46:602–5.

52. van Wassenaer-van Hall HN, van den Heuvel AG, Jansen GH, et al. Cranial MR in Wilson disease: abnormal white matter in extrapyramidal and pyramidal tracts. AJNR Am J Neuroradiol 1995;16:2021–7.

53. Piga M, Murru A, Satta L, et al. Brain MRI and SPECT in the diagnosis of early neurological involvement in Wilson's disease. Eur J Nucl Med Mol Imaging 2008; 35:716–24.

54. Page RA, Davie CA, MacManus D, et al. Clinical correlation of brain MRI and MRS abnormalities in patients with Wilson disease. Neurology 2004;63:638–43.

55. Sinha S, Taly AB, Prashanth LK, et al. Sequential MRI changes in Wilson's disease: with de-coppering therapy: a study of 50 patients. Neuroradiology 2006;48:613–21.

56. Strecker K, Schneider JP, Barthel H, et al. Profound midbrain atrophy in patients with Wilson's disease and neurological symptoms? J Neurol 2006;253: 1024–9.

57. Semnic R, Svetel M, Dragasevic N, et al. Magnetic resonance imaging morphometry of the midbrain in patients with Wilson disease. J Comput Assist Tomogr 2005;29:880–3.

58. Südmeyer M, Saleh A, Wojteckis L, et al. Wilson's disease tremor is associated with magnetic resonance imaging lesions in basal ganglia structures. Mov Disord 2006;21:2134–9.

59. Oder W, Prayer L, Grimm G, et al. Wilson's disease: evidence of subgroups derived from clinical findings and brain lesions. Neurology 1993; 43:120–4.

60. Hawkins RA, Mazziotta JC, Phelps ME. Wilson's disease studied with FDG and positron emission tomography. Neurology 1987;37:1707–11.

61. Hermann W, Barthel H, Hesse S, et al. Comparison of clinical types of Wilson's disease and glucose metabolism in extrapyramidal motor brain regions. J Neurol 2002;249:896–901.

62. Snow BJ, Bhatt M, Martin WR, et al. The nigrostriatal dopaminergic pathway in Wilson's disease studied with positron emission tomography. J Neurol Neurosurg Psychiatry 1991;54:12–7.

63. Cordato DJ, Fulham MJ, Yiannikas C. Pre-treatment and post-treatment positron emission tomographic scan imaging in a 20-year-old patient with Wilson's disease. Mov Disord 1998;13:162–6.

64. Barthel H, Hermann W, Kluge R, et al. Concordant pre- and postsynaptic deficits of dopaminergic neurotransmission in neurologic Wilson disease. AJNR Am J Neuroradiol 2003;24:234–8.

65. Jeon B, Kim J, Jeong JM, et al. Dopamine transporter imaging with [123I]-ß-CIT demonstrates presynaptic nigrostriatal dopaminergic damage in Wilson's disease. J Neurol Neurosurg Psychiatry 1998;65:60–4.

66. Walter U, Krolikowski K, Tarnacka B, et al. Sonographic detection of basal ganglia lesions in asymptomatic and symptomatic Wilson disease. Neurology 2005;64:1726–32.

67. Seeberger LC, Hauser RA. Cerebellar tremor. In: Lyons KE, Pahwa R, editors. Handbook of essential tremor and other tremor disorders. New York: Taylor and Francis; 2005. p. 227–41.

68. Bruberg JA, Jacquemont S, Hagerman RJ, et al. Fragile X premutation carriers characteristic MR imaging findings of adult male patients with progressive cerebellar and cognitive dysfunction. AJNR Am J Neuroradiol 2002;23(10):1757–66.

69. Bhatia KP, Schneider SA. Psychogenic tremor and related disorders. J Neurol 2007;254:569–74.

70. Bain PG, Aziz TZ, Liu X, et al. Deep brain stimulation. Oxford (UK): Oxford University Press; 2008.

Role of Transcranial Ultrasound in the Diagnosis of Movement Disorders

Jana Godau, MD*, Daniela Berg, MD

KEYWORDS

- Transcranial sonography • Parkinson's disease
- Movement disorders • Substantia nigra • Biomarker

Ultrasound of intracranial structures such as brain vessels or parenchyma through the intact skull was believed to be impossible until the 1980s. Since then, with ongoing improvements in the ultrasound technique, especially the development of transcranial color-coded sonography, ultrasound has gained increasing importance in the diagnosis of cerebrovascular disorders. In the early 1990s the first reports showed the possibility of differentiating main brain parenchymal structures sonographically in different parts of the brain, from the pontine brainstem to the parietal lobes, including the ventricular system and brainstem structures. With this method visualization of brain tumor tissue and cerebral hematomas was possible by ultrasound.[1–5] In 1995, Georg Becker and his group described for the first time a disease-specific sonographic finding in Parkinson disease (PD): hyperechogenicity of the substantia nigra (SN).[6] This finding began a new era of transcranial sonography. There had been no way of visualizing structural changes in PD using other structural neuroimaging techniques; this limitation in diagnosis was first challenged by the finding of the typical hyperechogenicity of the SN in PD.

Transcranial B-mode sonography (TCS) in movement disorders was met with scepticism from the scientific community, because it was hard to believe that a method for overcoming the acoustic bone window might show disease-specific abnormalities that could not be shown by other well-established structural neuroimaging methods. Since then, however, TCS results have been confirmed and extended by several independent groups internationally (see later discussion). TCS has become a reliable and valuable tool for the diagnosis and differential diagnosis of PD and other movement disorders. Because TCS is broadly available, quick to perform in moving patients, and inexpensive, it is worth considering as a supplementary diagnostic neuroimaging tool in general practice. This article provides a comprehensive summary on the ultrasound technique, the typical findings, and their value in the diagnosis and differential diagnosis of PD and other movement disorders.

TECHNIQUE: HOW TO PERFORM TCS

For TCS, a high-end ultrasound machine as applied in transcranial color-coded cerebrovascular ultrasound equipped with a 1.8- to 3.5-Mhz transducer should be used. An overview of the various systems that have been applied in studies is given in Table 1. Table 2 summarizes standard system settings from the authors' laboratory, which need to be individually optimized depending on the ultrasound system applied.

Scanning Procedure

The patient is in supine position, and the examiner usually sits at the head of the examination table. The examination is performed consecutively from each side, using the posterior or middle temporal

Department of Neurodegeneration, Center of Neurology and Hertie Institute for Clinical Brain Research, University of Tübingen, Hoppe-Seyler-Strasse 3, D-72076 Tübingen, Germany
* Corresponding author.
E-mail address: jana.godau@medizin.uni-tuebingen.de (J. Godau).

Neuroimag Clin N Am 20 (2010) 87–101
doi:10.1016/j.nic.2009.08.003
1052-5149/09/$ – see front matter © 2010 Elsevier Inc. All rights reserved.

Table 1
Ultrasound machines

	N	References
Advanced Technologies Laboratories (Washington, DC, USA)		
Ultramark 3000	1	7
Ultramark 9	1	8
General Electric (Milwaukee, WI, USA)		
Logiq 7	2	9, 10
Philips (Eindhoven, Netherlands)		
HDI 5000	2	11, 12
SONOS 4500	3	13–15
SONOS 5500	3	16–18
Siemens (Erlangen, Germany)		
Sonoline CF	3	6, 19, 20
Sonoline Elegra	35	21–56
Acuson Antares	1	57
Toshiba (Tokyo, Japan)		
SSH-140A	1	58
Aplio	1	59

Overview of the ultrasound systems that have been applied in studies (as current as Nov 2008). Manufacturers are given in alphabetical order. Number of publications (N) and references are given.

bone window. For evaluation of certain brain structures, including the mesencephalic brainstem, the basal ganglia, and the ventricle system, standardized axial scanning planes are used.[60] Several publications give detailed descriptions of the various brain structures and sonographical landmarks that can be depicted in these planes.[61–63]

To approach the plane of the mesencephalic brainstem, the ultrasound probe is placed at the temporal acoustic bone window in parallel to the imagined "orbitomeatal line" (**Fig.** 1A). In this plane, the butterfly-shaped structure of the mesencephalic brainstem, which is surrounded by the highly echogenic basal cisterns, can easily be delineated. Within the brainstem, several structures, including SN, red nucleus (RN), the brainstem midline raphe, and the aqueduct, can be visualized (**Fig.** 1D, E).

For evaluation of basal ganglia and ventricles, the ultrasound probe is slightly tilted 10° to 20° upwards with respect to the midbrain plane (see **Fig.** 1A). In this plane, the third ventricle, the anterior horn of the contralateral lateral ventricle and the anatomic site of the basal ganglia and the thalamus can be depicted (**Fig.** 1B, C). Structures close to the midline (SN, RN, raphe) are assessed at the side that is ipsilateral to the ultrasound probe. Structures more distant to the midline are assessed contralaterally to the probe.

Optimal tissue contrast and resolution may be achieved using the harmonic ultrasound reflections (tissue harmonic imaging, THI).[64] However, because this technique is more dependent on the quality of the acoustic bone window and is often limited concerning insonation depth, B-mode is

Table 2
System settings

Ultrasound transducer	1.8–3.5 MHz
Penetration depth	14–16 cm
Dynamic range	45–55 dB
Contour amplification	Medium–high
Postprocessing parameters	Moderate suppresion of low echo signals
Time gain compensation	Adjust as needed
Image brightness	Adjust as needed

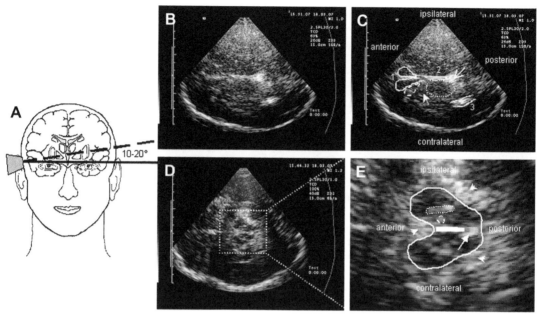

Fig. 1. Axial scanning planes. (*A*) The ultrasound probe is placed at the posterior or middle temporal bone window. The plane of the mesencephalic brainstem (*D, E*) is shown parallel to the orbitomeatal line (*continuous line*). When the probe is slightly tilted 10° to 20° upwards (*spaced line*) the plane of the third ventricle (*B, C*) can be visualized. (*B, C*) In the plane of the third ventricle, the ventricle system (*continuous lines*), including the anterior horns of the lateral ventricles (1), the third ventricle (2) and the posterior horn of the contralateral lateral ventricle with the echogenic choroid plexus (3) can be delineated. Contralaterally, the thalamus (*dotted line*), which is isoechogenic to the surrounding brain tissue, the slightly echogenic head of the caudate nucleus (*spaced line*), and the triangular anatomic area of the LN (*filled arrow*), which is normally isoechogenic to the surrounding brain tissue, can be seen. For better orientation the often highly echogenic pineal gland (*open arrow*) can be used. (*D, E*) In the plane of the mesencephalic brainstem, the butterfly-shaped hypoechogenic midbrain (*continuous line*), which is surrounded by the highly echogenic basal cisterns (*small arrows*), can be visualized easily. Within the brainstem, the echogenic structures of the ipsilateral SN (*dotted line*), RN (*spaced line*), and raphe (*thick line*) can be differentiated. The aqueduct is marked with an arrow.

required by convention for all quantitative and semiquantitative assessments (**Fig. 2**). Structures within the brainstem and the basal ganglia are denoted "hyperechogenic" when either the area (ie, of the SN) or the intensity (ie, hyperechogenicities in the basal ganglia) of the reflected signal are abnormally increased in contrast to the surrounding tissue. "Hypoechogenicity" is used to denote when the area or the intensity of the echogenic signal is abnormally decreased (ie, at the midline raphe).

Typical Sonographical Features

Mesencephalic brainstem
For clinical evaluation, assessment of the, in general, highly echogenic structures of SN, RN, and raphe within the hypoechogenic midbrain is essential.

SN The SN is a patchy or tie-shaped echogenic structure, visible bilaterally in the butterfly-shaped midbrain. The echogenic structure should be

visualized at its greatest extension to allow valid assessments. The extension can be biased by adjacent highly echogenic structures such as penetrating vessels or the RN, which need to be differentiated as clearly as possible. When the best depiction of the SN is achieved, the image is freezed and magnified 2- to 4-fold. For quantitative assessment the ipsilateral area of echogenicity of the SN is manually encircled with the cursor and its area is calculated automatically (compare **Fig. 1**E). SN hyperechogenicity is determined as an increased area of SN echogenicity, whereas SN hypoechogenicity is determined as diminished areas of SN echogenicity.

Cutoff values for increased and decreased SN echogenicity need to be established for each individual ultrasound system. SN areas of echogenicity above the 75th percentile of the normal population are classified as "moderately hyperechogenic," SN areas of echogenicity above the 90th percentile are classified as "markedly hyperechogenic" (**Fig. 3**). For the most frequently used ultrasound system in

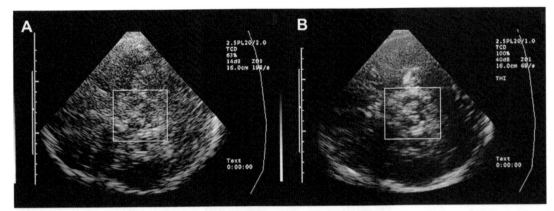

Fig. 2. Comparison of B-mode and THI. The contrast between the butterfly-shaped brainstem and the basal cisterns is higher in THI (*B*) compared with B-mode (*A*), as is the contrast between the midbrain tissue and the echogenic area at the anatomic site of the SN. Both images show SN hyperechogenicity; however, in (*B*) the SN appears larger, because its size is overestimated by the higher contrast using THI.

studies (Siemens Sonoline Elegra, Erlangen, Germany), cutoff values are 0.20 cm^2 for moderate and 0.25 cm^2 for marked hyperechogenicity.[21–23] Values less than 0.20 cm^2 are considered normal. SN hypoechogenicity is not yet clearly defined; however, several studies demonstrated SN hypoechogenicity when SN areas of echogenicity ranged below the 10th percentile.[9,24,25] Because of the limitations of resolution when small areas of SN echogenicity are assessed, values are normally given as sum values of both sides in the assessment of SN hypoechogenicity.

Raphe The highly echogenic brainstem midline structure represents the brainstem raphe. When the third ventricle is enlarged (see later discussion) the bottom of the third ventricle may be mistaken for the raphe. Therefore, scanning for raphe echogenicity should include the whole mesencephalic brain stem with special emphasis on the lower mesencephalon. The raphe is rated semiquantitatively using the echogenicity of either the RN or the basal cisterns as reference points.[6,19] Normally, the raphe constitutes a continuous highly echogenic line. When this line seems interrupted or not visible (ie, isoechogenic to the brainstem parenchyma) the raphe is classified as hypoechogenic (**Fig. 4**). The side of best visibility of the raphe is considered for assessment.

RN The RN is a highly echogenic round structure that normally appears as a small white dot posterior to the SN and lateral to the raphe. Neither a quantitative nor a semiquantitative rating has been standardized. In some publications, semiquantitative rating was performed by classifying the RN as hyperechogenic when either its area was enlarged or the echointensity was higher than in the basal cisterns.[25] RN hypoechogenicity has not been described. In the evaluation of movement disorders, RN assessment plays a minor role; however, the clear differentiation of RN and

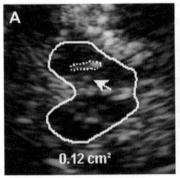
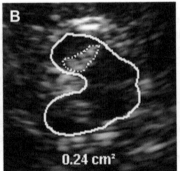
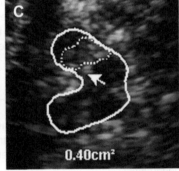

Fig. 3. SN hyperechogenicity. The midbrain is surrounded by the continuous line; the SN is manually encircled with a cursor on the side that is ipsilateral to the ultrasound probe (*dotted line*). It is important to differentiate the SN from the RN (*arrows, not visible in B*). (*A*) Normal SN echogenicity, (*B*) moderate SN hyperechogenicity, (*C*) marked SN hyperechogenicity.

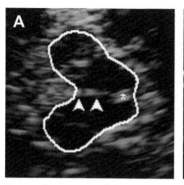
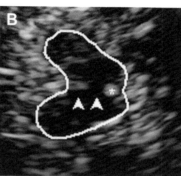
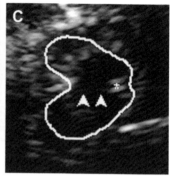

Fig. 4. Echogenicity of the raphe. The midbrain is surrounded by a continuous line, the echogenic midline raphe is marked with arrows. (A) Normal raphe echogenicity building a continuous line from the anterior surface to the aqueduct (*asterisk*). In (B) this line is interrupted; in (C) it is completely absent. Both conditions are defined as hypoechogenicity of the raphe.

SN, which can sometimes be challenging, is essential for the assessment of SN echogenicity (compare **Fig. 3**).

Third ventricle plane

The section through the thalami is reached by tilting the ultrasound probe 10° to 20° upwards when starting at the mesencephalic plane. For orientation, the usually calcified and therefore clearly depictable pineal gland generally indicates the correct plane.

Ventricle system As parts of the ventricle system in the third ventricle plane, the transverse diameter of the third ventricle and the transverse diameter of the contralateral anterior horn of the lateral ventricle can usually be measured (please compare **Fig. 5**).[65] The posterior horn of the lateral ventricle and the embedded choroid plexus can be visualized. Measurements are performed on the frozen and magnified (about twofold) images. To ensure reliable measurements of ventricle widths, diameters are measured between the inner surfaces of the surrounding hyperechogenic ependyma. These measurements are highly correlated with computed tomography (CT) assessments, although correlation is higher for the third ventricle ($r = 0.83$) than for the anterior horns of the lateral ventricles ($r = 0.73$), which may be attributed to the angulation of the probe.[65] Mean values for the ventricle widths have been shown to be 4.8 ± 1.9 mm (third ventricle) and 16.7 ± 2.3 mm (anterior horn of the lateral ventricle) for patients younger than 60 years. For elderly patients mean values are 7.6 ± 2.1 mm and 19.0 ± 2.9 mm respectively.[65]

Basal ganglia

In the same plane, the echogenicity of the contralateral thalamus, caudate nucleus, and lentiform nucleus (LN) can be assessed semiquantitatively.

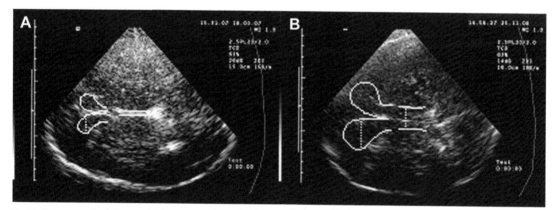

Fig. 5. Assessment of the ventricle system. Anterior horns of the ipsilateral and contralateral lateral ventricle and the third ventricle are marked with continuous lines. The sites of measurement for evaluation of ventricle widths are shown in dotted lines. (A) Normal width of the ventricle system. (B) Hydrocephalus with increased widths of the third ventricle and the lateral ventricles in a patient with aqueduct stenosis. In this image the septum pellucidum within the third ventricle can be seen.

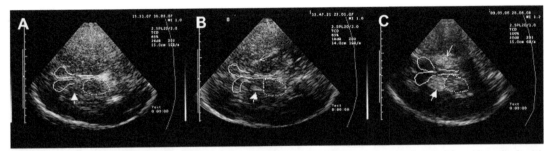

Fig. 6. Echogenicity of the LN. Anterior horns of the lateral ventricles and the third ventricle are marked with continuous lines (compare **Fig. 1**). The contralateral thalamus is marked with a dotted line. The contralateral anatomic area of the LN is marked with a filled arrow. (*A*) Normal LN echogenicity. The LN appears isoechogenic to the surrounding tissue. (*B*) LN hyperechogenicity in a patient with dystonia. LN hyperechogenicity can also be seen ipsilaterally (*small arrow*). (*C*) Massive bilateral LN hyperechogenicity in patient with Fahr disease. The anterior thalamus appears hyperechogenic.

Normally, these structures are isoechogenic to the surrounding brain parenchyma (grade 1). A moderate (grade 2) or marked (grade 3) hyperechogenicity is considered abnormal (please compare **Fig. 6**.[8,20] Similar to the assessment of SN echogenicity, quantitive evaluation of the echogenicity of the LN can be performed by manually encircling the area of increased echogenicity at its anatomic site and measuring the distances to the anterior horn and third ventricle.[20,26,62]

Causes of Echogenicity of Brain Structures

Generally, ultrasound echogenicity occurs at sites of great acoustic impedance difference between neighboring tissues, meaning that the ultrasound waves are reflected at tissue interfaces. Within single tissues echogenicity may result from a specific composition of neuronal, glial, and fiber components, as discussed for the brainstem midline raphe.[27] Alternatively, loads with heavy metals such as iron,[28,66] copper,[67] or manganese[67] may cause increased echogenicity of a certain brain structure. Changes of heavy metal content seem to be at least partly responsible for changes of echogenicity at the SN and the RN and for hyperechogenicity of the LN (ie, in dystonia).

The pathophysiologic conditions underlying changes of SN echogenicity are not fully understood. Hyperechogenicity of the SN is a typical sonomorphologic feature of idiopathic PD (iPD). Hypoechogenicity has primarily been demonstrated in restless legs syndrome (RLS). Both disorders have been associated with opposed alterations of SN iron content, leading to the suggestion that SN echogenicity is largely dependent on its iron content. Support for this hypothesis comes from several animal and postmortem studies that demonstrate a correlation of increased tissue iron concentration and SN hyperechogenicity[21,28,68–70] and from a study showing an association of SN hyperechogenicity and iPD with certain variants of the ceruloplasmin gene.[71] Ceruloplasmin is involved in the cellular iron influx and efflux. Three variations in the coding region of the gene that are associated with increased SN echogenicity and iPD have been described: Asp544Glu, Arg793His, and Ile63Thre. However, these changes account for only a small number of cases of SN hyperechogenicity. However, to date, increased tissue iron concentration is the only proven factor to have an impact on SN echogenicity. Further studies are needed to understand more comprehensively the biochemical conditions underlying SN echogenicity and its alterations.

Limitations

The main limitation of TCS is its dependency on the temporal acoustic bone window, allowing only partial or even no assessment of brainstem structures in some patients. The number of patients without insufficient bone windows varies between 5% and 60% depending on epidemiologic factors such as age and ethnicity.[13,14,24,29,59,72,73] It has been demonstrated that especially in elderly women bone windows may often be insufficient to allow full assessment of brainstem structures.[60] In white patients, temporal bone windows may allow only partial assessment of brainstem structures in 5% to 10% and of basal ganglia in 10% to 20% of patients.[60] In the Asian population difficulties with the bone windows may occur in 15% to 60% of patients.[13,14,59,72] No reports are available concerning the quality of temporal bone windows for TCS in Africans.

Another limitation is dependency of the method on the ultrasound system. Although most recent high-end ultrasound systems provide sufficient quality to allow reliable assessments of small echogenic structures in the brain, users are required to generate their own reference values, which account only for their own laboratory and system. Studies demonstrated considerable differences of absolute values for SN echogenicity, and even when using the same ultrasound system with identical system settings measurements may vary between 2 laboratories.[30] These minor differences can be of importance for multicenter scientific investigations, but do affect the daily routine examinations.

A third limitation of the method is its dependency on the experience and skill of the investigator.[11] In the authors' experience, however, an examiner who is experienced in other fields of B-mode or cerebrovascular ultrasound can be trained in TCS within 1 to 3 weeks. A completely inexperienced beginner may need up to 8 weeks to achieve sufficient skill. To allow broader application in the future, current research focuses on technological advances that may solve the problem of investigator dependency.

IMPLICATIONS: CLINICAL APPLICATION OF TCS

Despite the limitations of the method, a great number of studies demonstrate the value of TCS for the diagnosis and differential diagnosis of PD and other movement disorders. Because most research has been done on iPD, this article focuses on that disorder.

Role in PD

PD is the second most common movement disorder, which affects about 1% to 2% of the population older than 60 years. The diagnosis is based on the typical clinical symptoms, including bradykinesia, rigidity, resting tremor, and in later disease stages postural instability. Especially in the earlier disease stages when the clinical symptoms are less pronounced, it may be challenging to discriminate iPD from several other disorders, including atypical and symptomatic parkinsonian syndromes (aPS and sPS), essential tremor (ET) and depression with motor slowing. Typical symptoms determining aPS such as marked postural instability, vertical gaze palsy, and signs of frontal disinhibition in progressive supranuclear palsy (PSP) or marked autonomic dysfunction in multiple system atrophy (MSA-P) usually occur only later in the disease course. Therefore, distinction of these disorders at early disease stages is often not possible. This diagnostic uncertainty is reflected in a large postmortem study of 100 patients diagnosed with iPD during their lifetime by an experienced movement disorders specialist, which demonstrated the typical pathology (ie, Lewy bodies) in only 76% of patients.[74] Functional neuroimaging techniques assessing the function of the dopaminergic system improve the diagnostic certainty. Measurements include evaluation of a presynaptic dopaminergic deficit using mainly dopamine transporter imaging (DATScan) with single photon emission computed tomography (SPECT) and [^{123}I]β-CIT or [^{123}I]FP-CIT as tracers or positron emission tomography (PET) with the tracers [^{11}C]methylphenidate or [^{18}F]fluorodopa.[75–79] A primarily presynaptic dopaminergic deficit that is pronounced on one side generally indicates idiopathic PD. A primarily postsynaptic deficit as indicated by a decreased [^{123}I]iodobenzamide (SPECT) or [^{11}C]raclopride (PET) tracer uptake is usually associated with MSA-P or PSP. However, there is an overlap of pre- and postsynaptic neurodegeneration in both disease entities, making a clear diagnosis impossible in some cases. In later stages, structural magnetic resonance imaging (MRI) may show disease-specific abnormalities such as brainstem or frontal atrophy in PSP,[76,80,81] atrophy of the putamen and pontocerebellar fibers in MSA-P,[76,82,83] or unilateral cortical atrophy in corticobasal degeneration (CBD).[15] PET and SPECT examination have been shown to have good predictive values of more than 90% for the differentiation of ET and tremor-dominant iPD.[78,79,84,85]

However, although these imaging techniques demonstrate diagnostic parameters, their application is limited because of the high costs, invasiveness, and limited availability. Moreover, findings (especially functional neuroimaging findings) are not specific for a certain disease. In contrast, ultrasound is broadly available, quick to perform, inexpensive, noninvasive, and may differentiate between iPD and aPS (PSP, MSA-P) in most cases. The potential of TCS as an additional neuroimaging tool in the diagnosis and differential diagnosis of iPD, especially in the early disease stages, is discussed in the next section.

Differential diagnosis of iPD

The key finding in iPD is SN hyperechogenicity, which is present in more than 90% of patients, but only in up to 8% to 10% of healthy adults.[10,12,13,23,31,58,72] This could also be proven in a completely blinded study with the examination performed in a darkened room with patients completely covered with a sheet, so that the investigator could not be biased by unconcealable clinical features of PD like hypomimia or bradykinesia.[32] Moreover, SN hyperechogenicity not only allows differentiation of patients with iPD from healthy controls but also from patients with closely related disorders, such as the parkinsonian variant of MSA-P, PSP, ET, or depression.

aPS Several studies demonstrated good sensitivity and specificity of TCS for differentiation of iPD and aPS (Table 3). Results of 4 independent studies have shown that SN hyperechogenicity is only rarely found in MSA-P and in not more than one-third of PSP patients.[30,33,34,59] In addition to SN echogenicity, LN echogenicity (Fig. 5) and the width of the third ventricle (Fig. 6) can be determined. Typically, an iPD patient exhibits hyperechogenicity of the SN but normal echogenicity of the LN (positive predictive value 0.91), whereas a patient with MSA-P or PSP shows normal SN echogenicity along with hyperechogenicity of the LN (positive predictive value 0.96).[30,33,34] Assessment of the third ventricle may help to monitor brain atrophy, which is a typical additional feature in PSP.[34] Because all of these studies included patients after several years of disease, when the symptoms had progressed so far that the clinical diagnosis was obvious, the diagnostic value of TCS in early disease stages could not be determined. This gap was closed by a recently published prospective study of 60 patients presenting for the first time in a movement disorders specialist clinic with mild akinetic-rigid symptoms, which allowed a clinical diagnosis in accordance with the diagnostic criteria only in 37%.[29] In contrast, SN hyperechogenicity as a single parameter assessed at baseline allowed correct differentiation of iPD and aPS with good sensitivity (91%), specificity (82%), and positive predictive value (93%) when compared with the final clinical diagnosis and functional neuroimaging after 1 year. None of the patients with the final diagnosis of MSA-P or PSP showed SN hyperechogenicity. No additional gain in information could be observed by assessment of LN echogenicity in this study.

Some diagnostic blur may come from the rare disorders, dementia with Lewy bodies (DLB) and CBD, which have been shown to go along with SN hyperechogenicity in this and in prior studies.[35,36] Both disorders are known to show Lewy body pathology similar to iPD; however, an association of Lewy bodies and SN hyperechogenicity has not been found. As a result, TCS may distinguish iPD from MSA-P and PSP, but not from DLB or CBD, which, however, usually show unique clinical features already in very early disease stages. These data demonstrate that TCS is a helpful diagnostic tool in the diagnosis and differential diagnosis of PD even in early disease stages when differentiation by clinical features cannot be made.

Table 3
TCS in the differential diagnosis of iPD

TCS Finding	N	Indicated Condition	Excluded Condition	Sensitivity (%)	Specificity (%)	PPV (%)
SN hyperechogenicity	500[29,30,33,34,59]	iPD	aPS	92 (82–98)	80 (70–100)	91 (84–100)
Normal SN echogenicity	181[34]	MSA-P / MSA-P or PSP (<60 years)	iPD / iPD	90 / 75	98 / 100	86 / 100
Normal SN echogenicity plus LN hyperechogenicity	338[30,34]	MSA-P or PSP	iPD	57 (56–59)	99 (99–100)	98 (96–100)
Enlarged 3V (>10 mm) plus LN hyperechogenicity	181[34]	PSP	iPD	84	98	89

Pooled analysis. Values of single studies are given in brackets.
Abbreviations: 3V, third ventricle; PPV, positive predictive value.

ET TCS has been shown to differentiate tremor-dominant iPD from ET with a sensitivity of 75% to 86%, specificity of 84% to 93%, a positive predictive value of 91% to 95%.[10,85] However, the prevalence of SN hyperechogenicity in ET is 3 to 4 times higher than in healthy people.[10] In the literature, the risk of developing PD from ET is given as about 3 times higher compared with healthy controls.[86,87] In healthy individuals, SN hyperechogenicity is associated with a vulnerability of the nigrostriatal system (see later discussion). This association has led to the assumption that the increased prevalence of SN hyperechogenicity in ET may reflect the increased conversion rate to PD, suggesting that individuals with ET and SN hyperechogenicity have a higher risk of developing PD than individuals without this echo feature.[10] This hypothesis is currently being tested by several groups.

Depression Patients with depression often exhibit hypomimia, hypophonia, considerable motor slowing, and some increase in muscle tone, which may be difficult to distinguish from PD. However, similarly to ET, depression usually does not go along with SN hyperechogenicity, therefore this echo feature may be used for differentiation of both disorders. In depression, SN hyperechogenicity occurs about 2 to 3 times more often than in the general population.[37] Again, the conversion rate to PD is about 3 times higher in individuals with depression than in those without, suggesting that the ultrasound sign may reveal individuals at risk (see later discussion).[88,89] This hypothesis is supported by the finding that SN hyperechogenicity in depressed individuals is associated with mild motor asymmetry[37] and because depression constitutes a known premotor marker for iPD, which in retrospective studies has been observed several years before motor manifestation.[90,91]

Another sonographic feature that may help in the differential diagnosis of depression versus iPD is hypoechogenicity of the raphe. This echo feature is found in about 50% to 70% of individuals with unipolar depression and has been shown to be associated with responsivity to serotonergic medication.[19,37,38,92] However, raphe hypoechogenicity can also be found in 40% to 60% of iPD patients with depression[27,37,39] and in 63% of iPD patients with urge incontinence,[40] suggesting that neither SN echogenicity nor raphe echogenicity as single markers may reliably differentiate depression from iPD. However, in the clinical setting, when iPD and depression are suspected as differential diagnoses, the combination of normal SN echogenicity and hypoechogenicity of the raphe should indicate depression as the more likely diagnosis.

sPS TCS also allows differentiation of iPD and sPS, such as normal pressure hydrocephalus (NPH), welding-related parkinsonism, Wilson disease and Fahr disease. The enlargement of the ventricle system (see Fig. 6) as measured during the standard TCS procedure along with usually normal SN echogenicity can differentiate NPH from iPD. Metabolic disorders such as Wilson disease or Fahr disease and welding-related parkinsonism usually go along with marked hyperechogenicity of the basal ganglia (see Fig. 5), which can be attributed either to calcification or accumulation of heavy metals.[26,57] In Wilson disease the extent of LN hyperechogenicity correlates well with the clinical symptom severity, and even in asymptomatic patients some LN hyperechogenicity can be found.[26] Therefore visualization of the basal ganglia especially in unclear cases is important because several studies demonstrated that calcifications and trace metal depositions can be detected earlier with ultrasound than with cranial computed tomography (CCT) or MRI.[20,26,57] A definite diagnosis of vascular or posttraumatic parkinsonism with TCS is not possible, because underlying small basal ganglia lesions cannot be visualized.[14,41] However, even in these cases the absence of SN hyperechogenicity is valuable for the exclusion of iPD[14,41]:

Correlation of SN echogenicity and clinical features of iPD Several studies have shown the diagnostic potential of TCS in neurodegeneration. However, the causes underlying SN hyperechogenicity as the most specific feature of iPD and its pathophysiologic meaning are unclear. Several studies have tried to find associations between SN echogenicity and clinical features, certain PD subgroups, and the course of iPD to better understand SN hyperechogenicity as a biologic marker. Laterality of symptoms is a key feature of iPD. SN hyperechogenicity can usually be found bilaterally in iPD, although usually more pronounced contralaterally to the more affected side.[31,42] Marked laterality as measured by the laterality index (larger SN/smaller SN >1.15) can be found in 69% of iPD patients, but only in 20% of patients with DLB.[36] There are some differences between PD subtypes. For example, SN hyperechogenicity is less marked in tremor-dominant subtypes compared with akinetic-rigid forms of the disease.[42] In some forms of monogenetic PD (ie, caused by leucine-rich repeat kinase 2 [LRRK2] mutations) SN echogenicity is usually less prominent than in iPD, showing only borderline to moderate SN hyperechogenicity.[93] However, differences of iPD subtypes and monogenetic PD seem to be not marked enough to allow differential diagnosis. Regarding the impact of SN echogenicity on the disease course, greater SN hyperechogenicity was associated with younger age at motor symptom onset but with slower disease progression as measured by [^{18}F]fluorodopa PET.[42,43] In general, however, SN echogenicity seems to be a constant marker in adulthood, which does not change with age,[42–44] is constant in iPD patients for 5 years,[45] does not depend on the Hoehn and Yahr disease stage,[42,45] and does not correlate with dopaminergic function as assessed in SPECT examinations.[94] Regarding the differential diagnostic potential, TCS findings are consistent with the results of functional neuroimaging.[29,85] As a result, TCS is not useful as a marker for disease progression, but may allow diagnosis early in the disease course, when differentiation based on the clinical presentation may not be suggestive.

Premotor diagnosis of PD PD is a neurodegenerative disorder that is characterized by a progressive loss of dopaminergic cells. By the time of manifestation of first motor symptoms more than 50% of dopaminergic neurons are already lost.[95] Identification of individuals at risk for iPD in the premotor phase may form the basis for the establishment of effective neuroprotective treatment strategies.[90,91] SN hyperechogenicity is a stable marker that does not change with age in adulthood or with progression of iPD. Therefore, it seems a promising marker for iPD in early disease stages when clinical symptoms are not conclusive or potentially even before manifestation of motor symptoms. In the first published study on SN hyperechogenicity in iPD there were 2 healthy controls, who similarly to the iPD patients presented with SN hyperechogenicity. When 1 of these primarily healthy individuals developed PD only 2 years later (authors' unpublished data), a relation between SN hyperechogenicity and the putative risk of developing PD was discussed for the first time. Although results of prospective studies are not yet available, several studies demonstrate a strong association between SN hyperechogenicity and putative risk and premotor markers for iPD.

Association with epidemiologic risk factors for iPD In a large cohort of more than 800 healthy individuals it was shown that SN hyperechogenicity is correlated with male gender and a positive family history for iPD, both of which are known to be associated with an increased risk (about 4-fold) of developing iPD.[44] About 45% of first-degree relatives of iPD patients exhibit SN hyperechogenicity, suggesting an autosomal dominant inheritance of this sonographical marker.[96]

Association with vulnerability of the nigrostriatal system In monogenetic PD, asymptomatic mutation carriers exhibit SN hyperechogenicity similar to their relatives who already have the disease.[16] Asymptomatic carriers with reduced and normal presynaptic tracer uptake in PET examinations show SN hyperechogenicity, indicating that the ultrasound feature antecedes the dopaminergic cell loss, visualized by PET. Even in completely healthy individuals with SN hyperechogenicity, a slightly reduced tracer uptake in [^{18}F]fluorodopa PET can be observed, suggesting that a subclinical impairment of dopaminergic function might be related to SN hyperechogenicity.[21,28,46] SN hyperechogenicity is associated with slightly impaired motor function during demanding motor tasks even in young healthy people, as has been demonstrated, for example, in tap dancers with SN hyperechogenicity who experienced a "dead arm" while performing more often than their colleagues with normal SN echogenicity.[97] In neurodegeneratively healthy elderly people, SN hyperechogenicity is also associated with poorer motor performance.[22,73] In addition, cognitive performance in healthy individuals with SN hyperechogenicity seems to be slightly impaired, affecting visuospatial processing and sequential planning, which are primarily affected in iPD.[47] Following administration of neuroleptics, people with SN hyperechogenicity are more likely to develop parkinsonian symptoms, and to a more severe degree, than controls.[48] These findings imply that SN hyperechogenicity goes along with a certain vulnerability of the nigrostriatal system, which may progress to iPD in some individuals.

Association with putative premotor markers Retrospective examinations of iPD patients revealed several abnormalities that may antecede the onset of PD motor symptoms for several years. These abnormalities are named premotor symptoms and include, for example, olfactory dysfunction, REM sleep behavior disorder, depression, and autonomous symptoms such as constipation (for review see Ref.[90]). However, these symptoms are not specific to iPD and therefore do not allow the diagnosis. Several studies demonstrated that healthy individuals with reduced olfaction or depression exhibit SN hyperechogenicity and slightly impaired motor function significantly more often than controls.[37,49] However, the most evident argument for SN hypoechogenicity as a potentially premotor diagnostic marker is that at least 8 individuals who participated in various TCS studies as healthy controls and exhibited SN hyperechogenicity have developed PD, whereas the authors know of no cases of individuals with normal SN echogenicity developing PD (authors' yet unpublished data).

Prospective studies are needed to assess whether individuals with SN hyperechogenicity really have an increased risk of developing iPD. If this hypothesis was confirmed, TCS could serve as an excellent screening tool because of its broad availability, short duration, and low cost.

Role in Other Movement Disorders

Dystonia

Dystonia is characterized by a sustained contraction of muscles that interferes with motor control and may lead to distorted positions, which can affect 1 or several body parts or the whole body. In symptomatic forms of dystonia, which may result from vascular or metabolic lesions of the basal ganglia, CCT or MRI examinations may be conclusive for the disorder. However, differentiation of idiopathic dystonia, medication-induced dystonia, and psychogenic disorders mimicking dystonia may be more challenging, because normal CCT and MRI findings would be expected. TCS is a valuable tool for the diagnosis of upper-limb or cervical dystonia, demonstrating LN hyperechogenicity in more than 75% of patients.[20,50] In facial dystonia 31% of patients show LN hyperechogenicity, whereas in tardive dystonia or in psychogenic disorders, LN hyperechogenicity usually does not occur.[20,50] The pathophysiologic basis of LN hyperechogenicity in dystonia seems to be similar to that in Wilson disease, because in dystonia an association of LN hyperechogenicity and regional copper content and leukocyte copper metabolism was found.[67,98,99]

RLS

RLS has a prevalence of 5% to 15% and is one of the most common neurologic disorders, characterized by an irresistible urge to move the legs and sometimes other body parts, occurring at rest and generally relievable by moving around. Diagnosis is based on the patient's description of the typical symptoms, because especially in idiopathic RLS, clinical and neurologic examination, standard electrophysiologic assessment, CCT, and MRI show no abnormalities. TCS has demonstrated decreased SN echogenicity to allow diagnosis of RLS with a sensitivity of 82% and a specificity of 83% to 90%.[24,25] Sixty percent of patients with symptomatic RLS also exhibit SN hypoechogenicity.[24,25] In addition to decreased SN echogenicity, in more than 70% of patients with idiopathic RLS, hypoechogenicity of the brainstem raphe was found and increased echogenicity of the RN was found in about 60%, correlating with depression and periodic limb movements,

respectively.[25] Combined occurrence of 2 or more of these features indicated RLS with a positive predictive value of 97%. However, little is known about the value of TCS in the differential diagnosis of RLS. A first study of the differentiation of the comorbidity of RLS in a cohort of patients with polyneuropathy failed to show clinically significant differences in patients with polyneuropathy with or without RLS, although SN hypoechogenicity seemed to be associated with RLS (odds ratio 4.2).[100]

Other movement disorders

Only single reports exist on the diagnostic value of TCS for other movement disorders. In Huntington disease, increased echogenicity of the caudate nucleus is demonstrated.[8] In spinocerebellar ataxia, increased width of the fourth ventricle is found along with an often increased echogenicity of the dentate nucleus.[7] In spinocerebellar ataxia type 3, hyperechogenicity of the SN is demonstrated, reflecting the increased occurrence of mild PD symptoms in this disorder.[7] However, in none of these disorders does TCS provide more information than other neuroimaging techniques.

SUMMARY

Since its first application in PD in 1995, TCS has gained increasing attention and has been implemented in PD diagnosis internationally. TCS provides unique information that is supplementary to other structural or functional neuroimaging techniques. It has proved its potential in early and even preclinical diagnosis and differential diagnosis of PD, and its value in the diagnosis of other movement disorders. Regarding its quick and easy conduction, low cost, noninvasive nature, and broad availability, TCS is superior to other functional neuroimaging techniques such as PET and SPECT, which are used for the diagnosis and differential diagnosis of PD. Therefore it might be a useful instrument for general neurologists and for movement disorders specialists to add to their standard diagnostic workup. TCS may support a clinically suspected diagnosis of PD and may identify unclear cases who should be referred for functional neuroimaging. However, because TCS provides a stable marker, it cannot be used for determining progression of the disease. Taking into account the criteria of evidence classes I to IV as defined in a consensus report in accordance with criteria from the American Academy of Neurology (AAN),[60] results from several independent class II studies have shown the high predictive value of TCS in the differential diagnosis of iPD versus MSA-P and PSP (see **Table 3**). TCS reaches a level A recommendation in accordance with AAN criteria, and can therefore be recommended as a useful technique for the diagnosis and differential diagnosis of iPD.

REFERENCES

1. Becker G, Perez J, Krone A, et al. Transcranial color-coded real-time sonography in the evaluation of intracranial neoplasms and arteriovenous malformations. Neurosurgery 1992;31:420–8.
2. Becker G, Krone A, Koulis D, et al. Reliability of transcranial colour-coded real-time sonography in assessment of brain tumours: correlation of ultrasound, computed tomography and biopsy findings. Neuroradiology 1994;36:585–90.
3. Seidel G, Kaps M, Dorndorf W. Transcranial color-coded duplex sonography of intracerebral hematomas in adults. Stroke 1993;24:1519–27.
4. Maurer M, Becker G, Wagner R, et al. Early postoperative transcranial sonography (TCS), CT, and MRI after resection of high grade glioma: evaluation of residual tumour and its influence on prognosis. Acta Neurochir (Wien) 2000;142:1089–97.
5. Woydt M, Greiner K, Perez J, et al. Transcranial duplex-sonography in intracranial hemorrhage. Evaluation of transcranial duplex-sonography in the diagnosis of spontaneous and traumatic intracranial hemorrhage. Zentralbl Neurochir 1996;57: 129–35.
6. Becker G, Seufert J, Bogdahn U, et al. Degeneration of substantia nigra in chronic Parkinson's disease visualized by transcranial color-coded real-time sonography. Neurology 1995;45:182–4.
7. Postert T, Eyding J, Berg D, et al. Transcranial sonography in spinocerebellar ataxia type 3. J Neural Transm Suppl 2004;68:123–33.
8. Postert T, Lack B, Kuhn W, et al. Basal ganglia alterations and brain atrophy in Huntington's disease depicted by transcranial real time sonography. J Neurol Neurosurg Psychiatr 1999;67:457–62.
9. Schmidauer C, Sojer M, Seppi K, et al. Transcranial ultrasound shows nigral hypoechogenicity in restless legs syndrome. Ann Neurol 2005;58:630–4.
10. Stockner H, Sojer M, K KS, et al. Midbrain sonography in patients with essential tremor. Mov Disord 2007;22:414–7.
11. Skoloudik D, Fadrna T, Bartova P, et al. Reproducibility of sonographic measurement of the substantia nigra. Ultrasound Med Biol 2007;33:1347–52.
12. Ressner P, Skoloudik D, Hlustik P, et al. Hyperechogenicity of the substantia nigra in Parkinson's disease. J Neuroimaging 2007;17:164–7.
13. Huang YW, Jeng JS, Tsai CF, et al. Transcranial imaging of substantia nigra hyperechogenicity in a Taiwanese cohort of Parkinson's disease. Mov Disord 2007;22:550–5.
14. Tsai CF, Wu RM, Huang YW, et al. Transcranial color-coded sonography helps differentiation between idiopathic Parkinson's disease and vascular parkinsonism. J Neurol 2007;254:501–7.
15. Huang KJ, Lu MK, Kao A, et al. Clinical, imaging and electrophysiological studies of corticobasal degeneration. Acta Neurol Taiwan 2007;16:13–21.
16. Hagenah JM, Becker B, Bruggemann N, et al. Transcranial sonography findings in a large family with homozygous and heterozygous PINK1 mutations. J Neurol Neurosurg Psychiatr 2008;79:1071–4.
17. Hagenah JM, Konig IR, Becker B, et al. Substantia nigra hyperechogenicity correlates with clinical status and number of Parkin mutated alleles. J Neurol 2007;254:1407–13.
18. Hagenah JM, Hedrich K, Becker B, et al. Distinguishing early-onset PD from dopa-responsive dystonia with transcranial sonography. Neurology 2006;66:1951–2.
19. Becker G, Becker T, Struck M, et al. Reduced echogenicity of brainstem raphe specific to unipolar depression: a transcranial color-coded real-time sonography study. Biol Psychiatry 1995;38:180–4.
20. Naumann M, Becker G, Toyka KV, et al. Lenticular nucleus lesion in idiopathic dystonia detected by transcranial sonography. Neurology 1996;47: 1284–90.
21. Berg D, Becker G, Zeiler B, et al. Vulnerability of the nigrostriatal system as detected by transcranial ultrasound. Neurology 1999;53:1026–31.
22. Berg D, Siefker C, Ruprecht-Dorfler P, et al. Relationship of substantia nigra echogenicity and motor function in elderly subjects. Neurology 2001;56:13–7.
23. Walter U, Wittstock M, Benecke R, et al. Substantia nigra echogenicity is normal in non-extrapyramidal cerebral disorders but increased in Parkinson's disease. J Neural Transm 2002;109:191–6.
24. Godau J, Schweitzer KJ, Liepelt I, et al. Substantia nigra hypoechogenicity: Definition and findings in restless legs syndrome. Mov Disord 2007;22: 187–92.
25. Godau J, Wevers AK, Gaenslen A, et al. Sonographic abnormalities of brainstem structures in restless legs syndrome. Sleep Med 2008;9:782–9.
26. Walter U, Krolikowski K, Tarnacka B, et al. Sonographic detection of basal ganglia lesions in asymptomatic and symptomatic Wilson disease. Neurology 2005;64:1726–32.
27. Berg D, Supprian T, Hofmann E, et al. Depression in Parkinson's disease: brainstem midline alteration on transcranial sonography and magnetic resonance imaging. J Neurol 1999;246:1186–93.
28. Berg D, Roggendorf W, Schroder U, et al. Echogenicity of the substantia nigra: association with increased iron content and marker for susceptibility to nigrostriatal injury. Arch Neurol 2002;59: 999–1005.

29. Gaenslen A, Unmuth B, Godau J, et al. The specificity and sensitivity of transcranial ultrasound in the differential diagnosis of Parkinson's disease: a prospective blinded study. Lancet Neurol 2008;7:417–24.

30. Behnke S, Berg D, Naumann M, et al. Differentiation of Parkinson's disease and atypical parkinsonian syndromes by transcranial ultrasound. J Neurol Neurosurg Psychiatr 2005;76:423–5.

31. Berg D, Siefker C, Becker G. Echogenicity of the substantia nigra in Parkinson's disease and its relation to clinical findings. J Neurol 2001;248:684–9.

32. Prestel J, Schweitzer KJ, Hofer A, et al. Predictive value of transcranial sonography in the diagnosis of Parkinson's disease. Mov Disord 2006;21:1763–5.

33. Walter U, Niehaus L, Probst T, et al. Brain parenchyma sonography discriminates Parkinson's disease and atypical parkinsonian syndromes. Neurology 2003;60:74–7.

34. Walter U, Dressler D, Probst T, et al. Transcranial brain sonography findings in discriminating between parkinsonism and idiopathic Parkinson disease. Arch Neurol 2007;64:1635–40.

35. Walter U, Dressler D, Wolters A, et al. Sonographic discrimination of corticobasal degeneration vs progressive supranuclear palsy. Neurology 2004; 63:504–9.

36. Walter U, Dressler D, Wolters A, et al. Sonographic discrimination of dementia with Lewy bodies and Parkinson's disease with dementia. J Neurol 2006; 253:448–54.

37. Walter U, Hoeppner J, Prudente-Morrissey L, et al. Parkinson's disease-like midbrain sonography abnormalities are frequent in depressive disorders. Brain 2007;130:1799–807.

38. Walter U, Prudente-Morrissey L, Herpertz SC, et al. Relationship of brainstem raphe echogenicity and clinical findings in depressive states. Psychiatry Res 2007;155:67–73.

39. Becker T, Becker G, Seufert J, et al. Parkinson's disease and depression: evidence for an alteration of the basal limbic system detected by transcranial sonography. J Neurol Neurosurg Psychiatr 1997; 63:590–6.

40. Walter U, Dressler D, Wolters A, et al. Overactive bladder in Parkinson's disease: alteration of brainstem raphe detected by transcranial sonography. Eur J Neurol 2006;13:1291–7.

41. Kivi A, Trottenberg T, Kupsch A, et al. Levodoparesponsive posttraumatic parkinsonism is not associated with changes of echogenicity of the substantia nigra. Mov Disord 2005;20:258–60.

42. Walter U, Dressler D, Wolters A, et al. Transcranial brain sonography findings in clinical subgroups of idiopathic Parkinson's disease. Mov Disord 2006; 22:48–54.

43. Schweitzer KJ, Hilker R, Walter U, et al. Substantia nigra hyperechogenicity as a marker of predisposition and slower progression in Parkinson's disease. Mov Disord 2006;21:94–8.

44. Schweitzer KJ, Behnke S, Liepelt I, et al. Cross-sectional study discloses a positive family history for Parkinson's disease and male gender as epidemiological risk factors for substantia nigra hyperechogenicity. J Neural Transm 2007;114: 1167–71.

45. Berg D, Merz B, Reiners K, et al. Five-year follow-up study of hyperechogenicity of the substantia nigra in Parkinson's disease. Mov Disord 2005;20:383–5.

46. Walter U, Klein C, Hilker R, et al. Brain parenchyma sonography detects preclinical parkinsonism. Mov Disord 2004;19:1445–9.

47. Liepelt I, Wendt A, Schweitzer KJ, et al. Substantia nigra hyperechogenicity assessed by transcranial sonography is related to neuropsychological impairment in the elderly population. J Neural Transm 2008;115:993–9.

48. Berg D, Jabs B, Merschdorf U, et al. Echogenicity of substantia nigra determined by transcranial ultrasound correlates with severity of parkinsonian symptoms induced by neuroleptic therapy. Biol Psychiatry 2001;50:463–7.

49. Sommer U, Hummel T, Cormann K, et al. Detection of presymptomatic Parkinson's disease: combining smell tests, transcranial sonography, and SPECT. Mov Disord 2004;19:1196–202.

50. Becker G, Naumann M, Scheubeck M, et al. Comparison of transcranial sonography, magnetic resonance imaging, and single photon emission computed tomography findings in idiopathic spasmodic torticollis. Mov Disord 1997;12:79–88.

51. Becker G, Berg D, Lesch KP, et al. Basal limbic system alteration in major depression: a hypothesis supported by transcranial sonography and MRI findings. Int J Neuropsychopharmacol 2001;4:21–31.

52. Berg D, Hoggenmuller U, Hofmann E, et al. The basal ganglia in haemochromatosis. Neuroradiology 2000;42:9–13.

53. Godau J, Klose U, Di Santo A, et al. Multiregional brain iron deficiency in restless legs syndrome. Mov Disord 2008;23:1184–7.

54. Walter U, Horowski S, Benecke R, et al. Transcranial brain sonography findings related to neuropsychological impairment in multiple sclerosis. J Neurol 2007;254(Suppl 2):II49–52.

55. Niehaus LSN, Weber U. Brain parenchyma sonography in patients with essential tremor and Parkinson's disease. Cerebrovasc Dis 2004;17:3.

56. Behnke S, Berg D, Becker G. Does ultrasound disclose a vulnerability factor for Parkinson's disease? J Neurol 2003;250(Suppl 1):I24–7.

57. Walter U, Dressler D, Lindemann C, et al. Transcranial sonography findings in welding-related Parkinsonism in comparison to Parkinson's disease. Mov Disord 2008;23:141–5.

58. Kolevski G, Petrov I, Petrova V. Transcranial sonography in the evaluation of Parkinson disease. J Ultrasound Med 2007;26:509–12.

59. Okawa M, Miwa H, Kajimoto Y, et al. Transcranial sonography of the substantia nigra in Japanese patients with Parkinson's disease or atypical parkinsonism: clinical potential and limitations. Intern Med 2007;46:1527–31.

60. Walter U, Behnke S, Eyding J, et al. Transcranial brain parenchyma sonography in movement disorders: state of the art. Ultrasound Med Biol 2007;33: 15–25.

61. Berg D, Becker G. Perspectives of B-mode transcranial ultrasound. Neuroimage 2002;15:463–73.

62. Berg D, Behnke S, Walter U. Application of transcranial sonography in extrapyramidal disorders: updated recommendations. Ultraschall Med 2006;27:12–9.

63. Kern R, Perren F, Kreisel S, et al. Multiplanar transcranial ultrasound imaging: standards, landmarks and correlation with magnetic resonance imaging. Ultrasound Med Biol 2005;31:311–5.

64. Puls I, Berg D, Maurer M, et al. Transcranial sonography of the brain parenchyma: comparison of B-mode imaging and tissue harmonic imaging. Ultrasound Med Biol 2000;26:189–94.

65. Seidel G, Kaps M, Gerriets T, et al. Evaluation of the ventricular system in adults by transcranial duplex sonography. J Neuroimaging 1995;5:105–8.

66. Becker G, Berg D. Neuroimaging in basal ganglia disorders: perspectives for transcranial ultrasound. Mov Disord 2001;16:23–32.

67. Becker G, Berg D, Rausch WD, et al. Increased tissue copper and manganese content in the lentiform nucleus in primary adult-onset dystonia. Ann Neurol 1999;46:260–3.

68. Berg D, Hochstrasser H, Schweitzer KJ, et al. Disturbance of iron metabolism in Parkinson's disease – ultrasonography as a biomarker. Neurotox Res 2006;9:1–13.

69. Berg D, Grote C, Rausch WD, et al. Iron accumulation in the substantia nigra in rats visualized by ultrasound. Ultrasound Med Biol 1999;25:901–4.

70. Zecca L, Berg D, Arzberger T, et al. In vivo detection of iron and neuromelanin by transcranial sonography: a new approach for early detection of substantia nigra damage. Mov Disord 2005;20: 1278–85.

71. Hochstrasser H, Bauer P, Walter U, et al. Ceruloplasmin gene variations and substantia nigra hyperechogenicity in Parkinson disease. Neurology 2004;63:1912–7.

72. Kim JY, Kim ST, Jeon SH, et al. Midbrain transcranial sonography in Korean patients with Parkinson's disease. Mov Disord 2007;22:1922–6.

73. Behnke S, Double KL, Duma S, et al. Substantia nigra echomorphology in the healthy very old:

74. Hughes AJ, Daniel SE, Kilford L, et al. Accuracy of clinical diagnosis of idiopathic Parkinson's disease: a clinico-pathological study of 100 cases. J Neurol Neurosurg Psychiatr 1992;55:181–4.

75. Antonini A, Leenders KL, Vontobel P, et al. Complementary PET studies of striatal neuronal function in the differential diagnosis between multiple system atrophy and Parkinson's disease. Brain 1997; 120(Pt 12):2187–95.

76. Seppi K, Schocke MF, Esterhammer R, et al. Diffusion-weighted imaging discriminates progressive supranuclear palsy from PD, but not from the parkinson variant of multiple system atrophy. Neurology 2003;60:922–7.

77. Brooks DJ. Morphological and functional imaging studies on the diagnosis and progression of Parkinson's disease. J Neurol 2000;247(Suppl 2): II11–8.

78. Asenbaum S, Pirker W, Angelberger P, et al. [123I]beta-CIT and SPECT in essential tremor and Parkinson's disease. J Neural Transm 1998;105: 1213–28.

79. Benamer TS, Patterson J, Grosset DG, et al. Accurate differentiation of parkinsonism and essential tremor using visual assessment of [123I]-FP-CIT SPECT imaging: the [123I]-FP-CIT study group. Mov Disord 2000;15:503–10.

80. Brenneis C, Seppi K, Schocke M, et al. Voxel based morphometry reveals a distinct pattern of frontal atrophy in progressive supranuclear palsy. J Neurol Neurosurg Psychiatr 2004;75:246–9.

81. Warmuth-Metz M, Naumann M, Csoti I, et al. Measurement of the midbrain diameter on routine magnetic resonance imaging: a simple and accurate method of differentiating between Parkinson disease and progressive supranuclear palsy. Arch Neurol 2001;58:1076–9.

82. Brenneis C, Seppi K, Schocke MF, et al. Voxel-based morphometry detects cortical atrophy in the Parkinson variant of multiple system atrophy. Mov Disord 2003;18:1132–8.

83. Watanabe H, Saito Y, Terao S, et al. Progression and prognosis in multiple system atrophy: an analysis of 230 Japanese patients. Brain 2002; 125:1070–83.

84. Jennings DL, Seibyl JP, Oakes D, et al. (123I) beta-CIT and single-photon emission computed tomographic imaging vs clinical evaluation in Parkinsonian syndrome: unmasking an early diagnosis. Arch Neurol 2004;61:1224–9.

85. Doepp F, Plotkin M, Siegel L, et al. Brain parenchyma sonography and 123I-FP-CIT SPECT in Parkinson's disease and essential tremor. Mov Disord 2008;23:405–10.

correlation with motor slowing. Neuroimage 2007; 34:1054–9.

86. Zorzon M, Capus L, Pellegrino A, et al. Familial and environmental risk factors in Parkinson's disease: a case-control study in north-east Italy. Acta Neurol Scand 2002;105:77–82.

87. Koller WC, Busenbark K, Miner K. The relationship of essential tremor to other movement disorders: report on 678 patients. Essential Tremor Study Group. Ann Neurol 1994;35:717–23.

88. Schuurman AG, van den Akker M, Ensinck KT, et al. Increased risk of Parkinson's disease after depression: a retrospective cohort study. Neurology 2002; 58:1501–4.

89. Leentjens AF, Van den Akker M, Metsemakers JF, et al. Higher incidence of depression preceding the onset of Parkinson's disease: a register study. Mov Disord 2003;18:414–8.

90. Berg D. Marker for a preclinical diagnosis of Parkinson's disease as a basis for neuroprotection. J Neural Transm Suppl 2006;71:123–32.

91. Berg D. Biomarkers for the early detection of Parkinson's and Alzheimer's disease. Neurodegener Dis 2008;5:133–6.

92. Becker G, Struck M, Bogdahn U, et al. Echogenicity of the brainstem raphe in patients with major depression. Psychiatry Res 1994;55:75–84.

93. Schweitzer KJ, Brussel T, Leitner P, et al. Transcranial ultrasound in different monogenetic subtypes of Parkinson's disease. J Neurol 2007;254:613–6.

94. Spiegel J, Hellwig D, Mollers MO, et al. Transcranial sonography and [^{123}I]FP-CIT SPECT disclose complementary aspects of Parkinson's disease. Brain 2006;129:1188–93.

95. Fearnley JM, Lees AJ. Ageing and Parkinson's disease: substantia nigra regional selectivity. Brain 1991;114(Pt 5):2283–301.

96. Ruprecht-Dorfler P, Berg D, Tucha O, et al. Echogenicity of the substantia nigra in relatives of patients with sporadic Parkinson's disease. Neuroimage 2003;18:416–22.

97. Ruprecht-Dorfler P, Klotz P, Becker G, et al. Substantia nigra hyperechogenicity correlates with subtle motor dysfunction in tap dancers. Parkinsonism Relat Disord 2007;13:362–4.

98. Berg D, Weishaupt A, Francis MJ, et al. Changes of copper-transporting proteins and ceruloplasmin in the lentiform nuclei in primary adult-onset dystonia. Ann Neurol 2000;47: 827–30.

99. Kruse N, Berg D, Francis MJ, et al. Reduction of Menkes mRNA and copper in leukocytes of patients with primary adult-onset dystonia. Ann Neurol 2001;49:405–8.

100. Godau J, Manz A, Wevers AK, et al. Sonographic substantia nigra hypoechogenicity in polyneuropathy and restless legs syndrome. Mov Disord 2009;24:133–7.

Current Role of Functional MRI in the Diagnosis of Movement Disorders

Fatta B. Nahab, MD[a],*, Mark Hallett, MD[b]

KEYWORDS

* Neuroimaging * fMRI * Parkinson disease
* Tremor * Dystonia

The emergence of functional magnetic resonance imaging (fMRI) techniques for brain mapping has led to an explosion of data on normal brain physiology and the dysfunction that takes place with disease. This article provides a brief overview of fMRI methods and their applications in the study of neurologic movement disorders. There are today no clinical indications for the use of fMRI–based techniques in the area of neurologic movement disorders. We have therefore summarized seminal contributions in the various areas of movement disorder research, while providing a sketch of what this technology allows now and where this technology may lead.

HISTORY OF FUNCTIONAL NEUROIMAGING

Human interest in visualizing the active brain is nothing new. The notion that regional cerebral blood flow could serve as a surrogate marker of underlying neural activity was first demonstrated by the work of Roy and Sherrington in 1890.[1] Early efforts to map neural activity used short-lived radionuclides incorporated into compounds, such as glucose and water.[2,3] These radionuclides could be quantitatively and qualitatively measured with CT, leading to the development of positron emission tomography (PET).[4] The ongoing development of PET tracers has allowed for the virtually limitless ability to study any metabolic pathway, as

long as a relevant radiotracer could be synthesized to target the area of interest. The primary limitations associated with PET remain the radiation exposure, albeit limited; the extensive infrastructure required for synthesis of the radiopharmaceuticals; and lack of temporal resolution during data collection.

The development of MRI techniques for functional brain mapping is a much more recent development. A wide variety of techniques fall under the category of fMRI, with most techniques using the different magnetic properties of hydrogen atoms (protons) comprising water molecules ubiquitous throughout the body. Despite the lack of targeting probes as seen with PET, MR-based techniques compare favorably because of the availability of scanners at various points of care, lower cost of implementation, noninvasiveness, and higher temporal resolution compared with PET. However, no single imaging modality is likely to provide a comprehensive understanding; the use of complementary modalities in serial or parallel is now becoming a standard part of research protocols.

OVERVIEW OF fMRI TECHNIQUES

The technique most commonly used in fMRI studies is based on the principle of blood oxygen level–dependent (BOLD) contrast changes.[5]

[a] University of Miami Miller School of Medicine, 1120 NW 14th Street, Suite 1347 (C-215), Miami, FL 33136, USA
[b] Human Motor Control Section, Medical Neurology Branch, National Institute of Neurological Disorders and Stroke, NIH, Bethesda, MD, USA
* Corresponding author.
E-mail address: fnahab@med.miami.edu (F.B. Nahab).

Neuroimag Clin N Am 20 (2010) 103–110
doi:10.1016/j.nic.2009.08.001

BOLD-fMRI uses the different magnetic properties of oxygenated and deoxygenated hemoglobin to identify regional blood flow changes in the brain. If we assume a baseline level of neural activity and blood flow, then activation of this neural region will lead to increased oxygen consumption. This increased oxygen demand leads to a brief reduction (100–200 milliseconds) in the concentration of oxyhemoglobin relative to deoxyhemoglobin at the vascular bed. This small reduction in oxyhemoglobin is followed by a disproportionately larger compensatory increase in blood flow leading to an increase in oxyhemoglobin and drop in deoxyhemoglobin that surpasses preactivation levels. The signal from these blood flow changes is derived from the drop in deoxyhemoglobin, and leads to an increase in BOLD signal within a few seconds, which peaks around 4 to 8 seconds before it returns to baseline 14 to 16 seconds after the stimulus onset (Fig. 1).

Echoplanar imaging sequences are frequently used for these functional studies since they can rapidly collect multiple two-dimensional slice snapshots after the application of a single gradient radiofrequency pulse. With each slice being acquired in about 50 milliseconds, echoplanar imaging sequences can collect whole-brain volumes in a standard 2-second repetition time. Multiple volumes are collected during the course of a study.

fMRI EXPERIMENTAL DESIGNS

Based on the area of interest and the hypothesis, three main types of study designs are used in fMRI experiments: block, slow event-related, and fast event–related. Block design paradigms are the most frequently used because of their simplicity, ease of implementation, and sensitivity. This design consists of continuous presentation of a task for at least 20 seconds followed by an alternate condition, frequently a rest period of similar duration. The data collected from a block design experiment allow each task condition to be averaged to improve the signal-to-noise ratio (SNR) and then a simple "contrast" can be performed to compare the two conditions. The contrast can be as simple as a subtraction of the BOLD responses of one condition from another or, more commonly, parametric statistics are performed at each voxel (Fig. 2).

The prolonged duration required for each condition in a block design experiment, however, has many inherent design limits. For example, the long duration required for each condition limits the ability to study multiple conditions within the time constraints of a standard scanning session. The ability to extract temporal information about the brain responses is also limited because of the prolonged BOLD response. These restrictions among others have led to the use of slow and fast event–related designs. In the case of slow event–related paradigms, the standard experimental blocks are shortened while maintaining the alternating patterns of stimulation. Fast event–related experiments, on the other hand, consist of rapid stimulus periods (as short as 34 milliseconds) occurring repeatedly at varying intervals. All of these experimental designs assume a linearity with the BOLD signal,[6] with fast event–related designs being most dependent on this principle. Despite the apparent advantages associated with the faster designs, each sacrifices some SNR (35% drop in SNR for slow event–related vs block[7]; 17%–25% drop in SNR for fast event–related vs slow event–related[8]), though this is arguably outweighed by the increased number of trials possible.

fMRI DATA ANALYSIS

A detailed summary of the various steps required to process fMRI data is beyond the scope of this review. For those interested in learning more about

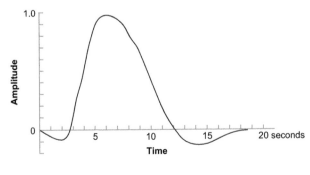

Fig. 1. Predicted BOLD hemodynamic response function following a brief stimulus. The hemodynamic response function demonstrates the three characteristic regions: the initial dip, the rising phase, and the poststimulus undershoot. The significance of the initial dip has been shown to represent the early increased oxygen consumption and increase in deoxyhemoglobin before the blood flow response. The rising phase reflects the lagging contribution of the blood flow response, which leads to an overcompensation (peak) whereby deoxyhemoglobin concentrations are even below baseline levels. This drop in deoxyhemoglobin leads to the increase in signal intensity. The mechanisms behind the poststimulus undershoot are not well understood and vary by task.

Predicted BOLD Response by Study Design

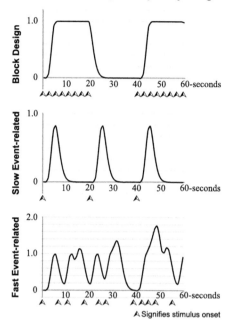

A Signifies stimulus onset

Fig. 2. Overview of fMRI–based paradigm designs. A standard block design demonstrates the expected prolonged BOLD response with a continuous stimulus or task performance alternating with periods of rest, leading to a change from the task-specific BOLD response. Slow event–related designs allow more frequent stimulus presentations while still allowing a complete separation of BOLD response among potentially different stimuli. Fast event–related responses are presented in a random or pseudo-random manner. This generates a BOLD response, which cannot be easily resolved without analytical tools, such as deconvolution, to separate the contributions of each respective task over time.

the various steps in preprocessing and data analysis at the single subject and group level, we recommend "Functional Imaging Analysis Contest (FIAC) Analysis According to AFNI and SUMA," by Z.S. Saad and colleagues (Hum Brain Mapp 2006;27:417–24).

CLINICAL INDICATIONS OF fMRI TO DIAGNOSE NEUROLOGIC MOVEMENT DISORDERS

The rapid development of fMRI for both clinical and nonclinical applications provides a unique opportunity to use this exciting modality for answering questions related to pathophysiology and diagnostic uncertainty, for identifying mechanisms of therapeutic action, and for monitoring effectiveness of therapy, among many other tasks. Despite the wide array of opportunities for the use of fMRI as a clinical test, no indications are

currently available for its use in neurologic movement disorders. The following sections provide an overview of the large volume of work that has taken place in this area, and points to potential directions for future clinical applications.

SUMMARY OF fMRI FINDINGS IN SELECT MOVEMENT DISORDERS
Parkinson Disease

Clinical overview of Parkinson disease
Parkinson disease was first described in 1817 by James Parkinson in "An Essay on the Shaking Palsy." Parkinson disease is the second most common neurodegenerative disorder, after Alzheimer disease, with a prevalence of 0.6%. The clinical hallmarks of Parkinson disease include:

Resting tremor
Muscle rigidity
Bradykinesia
Postural instability

At least two of these aforementioned features are required to make a formal diagnosis, though the symptoms of Parkinson disease include a diverse range of other motor and nonmotor impairments. Many of these impairments are attributed to a loss of dopaminergic cells in the substantia nigra, which project from the midbrain to such areas as the putamen and caudate in the striatum. Since the predominant abnormality in Parkinson disease involves a loss of dopamine production, therapy is targeted at restoring dopamine levels. Dopamine levels can be increased using a wide variety of approaches, including the use of dopamine precursors (levodopa) converted to dopamine by the brain, the use of dopamine agonists, or by slowing the breakdown or reuptake of dopamine at nerve terminals.

The constellation of clinical features combined with evidence of a functional improvement on dopaminergic therapy helps to confirm the diagnosis of primary or idiopathic Parkinson disease. Idiopathic Parkinson disease is the most common parkinsonism, accounting for 42% of cases.[9] However, many varieties of parkinsonisms present with distinctive combinations of clinical findings and a lack of response to dopaminergic therapy. These dopamine-nonresponsive disorders are referred to as Parkinson-plus syndromes and include multiple system atrophy, progressive supranuclear palsy, and corticobasal degeneration. As a group, Parkinson-plus disorders progress more rapidly than primary or secondary parkinsonisms and have more widespread and severe neuro-degeneration. A review of each of these disorders and their similarities or differences is beyond the scope of this review, though the current best in vivo method for differentiating between primary, secondary, and Parkinson-plus disorders is a clinical examination by an experienced movement disorder neurologist. Furthermore, the distinctive characteristics of these various disorders frequently become evident only after a diagnosis of parkinsonism is made and treatments are found to be ineffective. Such limitations in early diagnosis constrain the ability of the clinician to develop a stratified plan of management based on the particular disease subtype.

fMRI studies of Parkinson disease

Early fMRI studies of Parkinson disease aimed to identify differences between patients and controls in the motor network. Such differences, it was hoped, could be used as signatures of the disorder. Early work by Tada[10] noted decreased activation in the supplementary motor area during movement in Parkinson disease versus controls. This finding was confirmed by Sabatini and colleagues,[11] who also demonstrated a common pattern of motor network activation (premotor, motor, parietal cortex, striatum, and cerebellum) in both groups, though cortical motor areas showed higher levels of activation in patients than in controls. Similar findings were reported using PET[12,13] and single photon emission CT (SPECT),[14] while others[15,16] found reduced activation in motor-related cortical areas. These seemingly discrepant findings are disconcertingly common in the neuroimaging literature. It should be noted, however, that these findings emphasize the context-specific performance of the neural networks being studied. In the majority of these neuroimaging studies, efforts were made to ensure that state-related confounds (eg, differing performance, effort, anxiety) were minimized among the groups being compared. Despite such efforts, it is inevitable that such confounds exist even in patients with mild disease when compared with healthy controls.

The cognitive manifestations of Parkinson disease have also been studied with fMRI. The findings of these early studies have identified dysfunction in numerous cognitive domains, including working memory,[17] set-shifting or the ability to alter behavior to dynamically changing circumstances,[18] reward processing,[19] and semantic sequencing.[20] Such cognitive impairments also have the potential to affect motor performance. This was evident when subjects with Parkinson disease performed both simple and complex dual tasks during fMRI.[21] The findings suggested that poorer performance of dual tasks related to impairments in attention,

impairments in performance monitoring, and a limited capacity of such resources. Despite the behavioral basis of these impairments, administration of a dopaminergic agent led to both an enhancement of prefrontal cortex performance, relative to a baseline hypodopaminergic state, and normalization of fMRI activation patterns.[22]

The development of a noninvasive measure to distinguish the various parkinsonian subtypes might also serve as a tool to monitor disease progression and the impact of therapy. Work by a number of groups using fMRI as a potential biomarker to differentiate disease subtypes and to monitor progression is ongoing. No clinical indications are yet approved for the use of fMRI in patients suspected of having parkinsonism.

Dystonia

Dystonia is a neurologic movement disorder characterized by sustained muscle contractions that lead to disabling repetitive movements or abnormal postures. Dystonia can begin at any age from childhood through late adulthood. Early-onset cases (before the age of 25), referred to as *primary dystonia*, typically present with a generalized pattern of muscle involvement and can lead to disabling muscular and orthopedic deformities. Patients with a later onset of dystonia typically present with more focal or segmental regions of involvement, with the most common presentation being cervical dystonia. The prevalence of primary generalized dystonia is estimated to be 3.4 per 100,000, while the frequency of focal dystonias is 29.5 per 100,000.[23]

The etiologic mechanisms of dystonia are not known and no test is currently available for diagnostic confirmation, with exception of a small number of inherited subtypes (eg, *DYT-1* mutation) confirmed by genetic testing. One possible cause of dystonic symptoms involves neurotransmitter changes that lead to an imbalance of dopamine transmission within the basal ganglia.[24,25] Direct evidence for this comes from dopa-responsive dystonia. Indirect evidence for this hypothesis comes from the development of dystonic symptoms in patients treated with the dopamine precursor levodopa (used to treat Parkinson disease) or following the use of dopamine antagonists frequently used to treat psychosis. Additionally, observations of patients with dystonia note difficulty initiating and performing voluntary movements using only the appropriate muscles required to carry out the action. In such cases, antagonist muscles are simultaneously activated, leading to muscular "co-contraction" and the appearance of dystonic sustained muscular contractions.

This observation has led to the hypothesis that normal brain mechanisms leading to the inhibition of surrounding antagonist muscles are impaired in dystonia.

Routine structural imaging of the brain in patients suspected of having dystonia show no consistent abnormalities. Studies using diffusion tensor imaging to characterize the architectural integrity of white matter tracts have identified changes in subgyral sensorimotor cortex[26] and the lentiform nucleus,[27] with the latter area appearing to normalize 4 weeks after treatment with botulinum toxin.[28] Voxel-based morphometry methods have similarly been useful in identifying subtle changes in the gray matter volumes of subjects with dystonia.[29,30]

Functional imaging methods, such as PET and fMRI, have provided additional insights into the neural mechanisms underlying dystonia. Abnormalities in premotor, supplementary motor, and primary motor cortices have been identified during movement in both generalized and focal dystonias. These results are confusing because one study showed decreased activity of patients relative to controls,[31] and other studies showed increased activity.[32,33] Future studies would likely benefit from the inclusion of behavioral measures, such as electromyography during fMRI, to allow for better differentiation of task from rest, while matching performance with healthy controls.[34]

Essential Tremor

Essential tremor, a common movement disorder, is seen as early as childhood with increasing incidence with age. It affects up to 14% of people over age 65. Essential tremor is most frequently exemplified by rhythmic shaking of the arms, but may also involve the head, tongue, legs, voice, and face. Essential tremor is recognized as a heritable disorder with apparent Mendelian autosomal dominant transmission, though no disease-causing genes have yet been clearly identified. Treatments are based primarily on pharmacologic agents, although surgical intervention may be an option in the most disabling cases.

The pathophysiology of essential tremor has been only partially defined. A number of direct and indirect neurophysiological studies have implicated a neuronal network involving the thalamus, the sensorimotor cortex, the inferior olivary nuclei, and cerebellum in the production of essential tremor. This is also supported by an animal model using harmaline, which induces a reversible essential tremor–like state with abnormal tremor-specific oscillations observed in the olivocerebellar pathway.

Studies of essential tremor using fMRI have helped to confirm the neural network involved. Such studies have typically contrasted the brain activations observed during postural or action tremors in essential tremor patients with the brain responses of patients during rest when the tremor resolves, or with healthy controls mimicking tremor. Findings from a number of studies[35,36] have consistently shown involvement of a widespread motor network associated with tremor, including primary motor cortex, primary sensory cortex, thalamus, globus pallidus, red nucleus, cerebellar hemispheres, and dentate nucleus of the cerebellum. Mimicked tremor by healthy controls led to a similar network becoming active, though at slightly lower levels than in patients. These findings suggest that tremor is generated through the same neural network that generates voluntary movement. Studies to date, however, have been unable to elucidate the location of the tremor oscillations. Determining whether there are changes in functional connectivity may also help to explain the occurrence of the tremor during posture or action, but not at rest.

Studies in essential tremor give some indication about the difficulties in this sort of work. Studies at rest in the patients seem theoretically fair to compare in the treated and untreated condition, and even to compare with normals. However, tremor is not present in this situation. Studies with voluntary movement and tremor are difficult to compare with normal voluntary movement, even if tremor is mimicked.

Huntington Disease

Huntington disease is a hereditary progressive neurodegenerative disorder with neurologic and psychiatric features. The classic signs of Huntington disease include the development of chorea (diffuse, involuntary, rapid, irregular, jerky movements) and a gradual loss of thought processing and acquired intellectual abilities (dementia). Although symptoms typically become evident during the fourth or fifth decades of life, the age at onset is variable and ranges from early childhood to late adulthood (eg, 70s or 80s). Huntington disease is transmitted has an autosomal dominant inheritance pattern, with disease severity and age of onset correlating with the number of trinucleotide DNA repeats on chromosome 4. The neuro-degeneration associated with Huntington disease primarily affects the basal ganglia (especially the caudate nucleus) and the cerebral cortex.

The use of fMRI to study Huntington disease has primarily focused on two goals: characterizing the neural dysfunction and developing a biomarker for presymptomatic diagnosis. To assess the impact of Huntington disease on various neural domains, performance of functional tasks was assessed during fMRI and compared with that of healthy controls. Huntington disease patients were found to have widespread cortical and subcortical increased BOLD responses on maze perfor-mance[37] and the Simon effect task,[38] especially in motor and visual processing areas. A lack of motor response inhibition also correlates with patterns of impaired activation in the caudate and thalamus.[39] The constellation of fMRI changes in activation and connectivity[40] suggests that the neuro-degeneration or decreased activation observed in basal ganglia leads to compensatory recruitment (hyperactivation) of accessory motor pathways.[41]

The development of a biomarker to predict the onset of Huntington disease in the presymptom-atic stage is critical to improvements in disease management. Efforts to develop such a test based on the fMRI patterns previously described have led to a variety of potential measures, though further work is needed to validate these findings before clinical implementation can proceed. The task-related patterns of basal ganglia hypoactivation noted in symptomatic disease are preceded by a period of increased activation in the caudate, thalamus, and frontotemporal cortices,[42] which likely signifies local compensation taking place in the setting of early neuro-degeneration. Activation of the left dorsal anterior insula during the process-ing of disgusted facial expressions was also absent in Huntington disease.[43] These and numerous other changes on fMRI have been able to identify presymptomatic Huntington disease as early as 12 years before the estimated disease onset.[44] Despite these promising results, it should be noted that all studies to date have reported these differences at the group level. Because of the high degree of variability inherent in presymp-tomatic Huntington disease, assessing risk of future disease at the single subject level is not currently possible.

FUTURE DIRECTIONS FOR fMRI

The utility of fMRI in the field of neurologic move-ment disorders is only in its infancy. The early find-ings we have summarized thus far have adopted traditional case-control visual comparisons of statistical parametric maps. Furthermore, the vast majority of studies used block-design para-digms with alternating periods of rest and tasks with limited ecological validity. Attempts in most studies were made to minimize confounds between patients and controls, though in our view these efforts have only skimmed the surface and may explain many of the differences identified between patients and controls. For example, when we look at the neural correlates of essential tremor, we find no qualitative differences in brain activation identified by fMRI between patients with tremor and subjects simulating tremor. What is most commonly identified is a quantitative differ-ence in activation with unknown clinical or physio-logic significance. Such small quantitative differences may even be a consequence of subtle asymmetries in performance between patients and controls. Having identified the potential weak-nesses of fMRI–based methods in neurologic movement disorders, we would now like to high-light the unique contributions this modality can provide.

Advances in the speed and quality of higher field-strength MRI hardware, and the development of a wealth of methods to more fully characterize the BOLD response, have greatly stimulated the growth of fMRI in clinical research over the past decade. Studies comparing activation maps between patients and controls are now comple-mented by measures of functional connectivity to characterize the actions of the neural network at large. These developments are being enhanced further with the ability to simultaneously collect both high spatial-resolution fMR image–based BOLD responses and high temporal-resolution electroencephalography. More recently, transcra-nial magnetic stimulation performed during fMRI has allowed investigators to understand the impact of a virtual lesion both locally and on the neural network. The use of a combination of MR modalities, such as MR spectroscopy or diffusion tensor imaging, helps to provide a comprehensive understanding of the pathologic changes not seen by standard structural MR imaging sequences.

Newer methods of BOLD-fMRI analysis will also make a significant impact on our understanding of the brain. Older univariate methods of analysis have limited sensitivity because they depend on restricted models of the BOLD response. These sensitivity limits drive the need for longer studies, which would collect adequate amounts of data but would also increase the risk of inducing patient fatigue. With the development of more sophisti-cated statistical methods and with the reduction in costs of high-throughput computing, multivar-iate analyses of fMRI data can now be performed relatively quickly. Model-based analyses are being replaced by "artificial intelligence" or "machine learning" methods, which are model independent. These more sophisticated techniques are also providing the statistical power necessary to make inferences on brain activations collected over just a few seconds. Rapid acquisition and interpretation now allows the MR image scanner to provide the participant with near–real-time biofeedback of their brain responses.

Thanks largely to the availability, sensitivity, and non-invasiveness of fMRI, clinical and non-clinical applications for the modality have rapidly emerged. The use of fMRI to probe brain function in neurologic movement disorders is only in its infancy.

REFERENCES

1. Roy C, Sherrington C. On the regulation of the blood supply of the brain. J Physiol 1890;11:85–108.
2. Reivich M, Kuhl D, Wolf A, et al. Measurement of local cerebral glucose metabolism in man with 18F-2-fluoro-2-deoxy-d-glucose. Acta Neurol Scand Suppl 1977;64:190.
3. Huang SC, Carson RE, Hoffman EJ, et al. Quantitative measurement of local cerebral blood flow in humans by positron computed tomography and 15O-water. J Cereb Blood Flow Metab 1983;3(2):141–53.
4. Ter-Pogossian MM, Phelps ME, Hoffman EJ, et al. A positron-emission transaxial tomograph for nuclear imaging (PETT). Radiology 1975;114(1):89–98.
5. Ogawa S, Lee T, Nayak A, et al. Oxygenation-sensitive contrast in magnetic resonance image of rodent brain at high magnetic fields. Magn Reson Med 1990;14:68–78.
6. Boynton GM, Engel SA, Glover GH, et al. Linear systems analysis of functional magnetic resonance imaging in human V1. J Neurosci 1996;16(13): 4207–21, ISSN: 02706474.
7. Bandettini PA, Cox RW. Event-related fMRI contrast when using constant interstimulus interval: theory and experiment. Magn Reson Med 2000;43(4): 540–8, ISSN: 07403194.
8. Miezin FM, Maccotta L, Ollinger JM, et al. Characterizing the hemodynamic response: effects of presentation rate, sampling procedure, and the possibility of ordering brain activity based on relative timing. Neuroimage 2000;11(6):735–59, ISSN: 10538119.
9. Bower JH, Maraganore DM, McDonnell SK, et al. Incidence and distribution of parkinsonism in Olmsted County, Minnesota, 1976–1990. Neurology 1999;52(6):1214–20, ISSN: 00283878.
10. Tada Y. [Motor association cortex activity in Parkinson's disease–a functional MRI study]. Rinsho Shinkeigaku 1998;38(8):729–35 [in Japanese].
11. Sabatini U, Boulanouar K, Fabre N, et al. Cortical motor reorganization in akinetic patients with Parkinson's disease: a functional MRI study. Brain 2000; 123:394–403.
12. Brooks DJ. Functional imaging of Parkinson's disease: is it possible to detect brain areas for specific symptoms? J Neural Transm Suppl 1999; 56:139–53, ISSN: 03036995.
13. Catalan MJ, Ishii K, Honda M, et al. A PET study of sequential finger movements of varying length in patients with Parkinson's disease. Brain 1999; 122(3):483–95, ISSN: 00068950.
14. Rascol O, Sabatini U, Fabre N, et al. The ipsilateral cerebellar hemisphere is overactive during hand movements in akinetic parkinsonian patients. Brain 1997;120(1):103–10, ISSN: 00068950.
15. Playford ED, Jenkins IH, Passingham RE, et al. Impaired mesial frontal and putamen activation in Parkinson's disease: a positron emission tomography study. Ann Neurol 1992;32(2):151–61, ISSN: 03645134.
16. Jahanshahi M, Jenkins IH, Brown RG, et al. Self-initiated versus externally triggered movements—I. An investigation using measurement of regional cerebral blood flow with PET and movement-related potentials in normal and Parkinson's disease subjects. Brain 1995;118(4):913–33, ISSN: 00068950.
17. Lewis SJ, Dove A, Robbins TW, et al. Cognitive impairments in early Parkinson's disease are accompanied by reductions in activity in frontostriatal neural circuitry. J Neurosci 2003;23(15):6351–6.
18. Monchi O, Petrides M, Doyon J, et al. Neural bases of set-shifting deficits in Parkinson's disease. J Neurosci 2004;24(3):702–10.
19. Schott BH, Niehaus L, Wittmann BC, et al. Ageing and early-stage Parkinson's disease affect separable neural mechanisms of mesolimbic reward processing. Brain 2007;130:2412–24 [Epub 2007 Jul 11].
20. Tinaz S, Schendan HE, Stern CE. Fronto-striatal deficit in Parkinson's disease during semantic event sequencing. Neurobiol Aging 2008;29(3):397–407 [Epub 2006 Dec 8].
21. Wu T, Hallett M. Neural correlates of dual task performance in patients with Parkinson's disease. J Neurol Neurosurg Psychiatr 2008;79(7):760–6, ISSN: 00223050.
22. Fera F, Nicoletti G, Cerasa A, et al. Dopaminergic modulation of cognitive interference after pharmacological washout in Parkinson's disease. Brain Res Bull 2007;74(1–3):75–83 [Epub 2007 Jun 6].
23. Nutt JG, Muenter MD, Aronson A, et al. Epidemiology of focal and generalized dystonia in Rochester, Minnesota. Mov Disord 1988;3:188–94, ISSN: 08853185.
24. Wooten GF, Eldridge R, Axelrod J, et al. Elevated plasma dopamine-beta-hydroxylase activity in autosomal dominant torsion dystonia. N Engl J Med 1973;288(6):284–7, ISSN: 00284793.
25. Furukawa Y, Hornykiewicz O, Fahn S, et al. Striatal dopamine in early-onset primary torsion dystonia with the DYT1 mutation. Neurology 2000;54(5): 1193–5, ISSN: 00283878.

26. Carbon M, Kingsley PB, Su S, et al. Microstructural white matter changes in carriers of the DYT1 gene mutation. Ann Neurol 2004;56(2):283–6, ISSN: 03645134.

27. Colosimo C, Pantano P, Calistri V, et al. Diffusion tensor imaging in primary cervical dystonia. J Neurol Neurosurg Psychiatr 2005;76(11):1591–3, ISSN: 00223050.

28. Blood AJ, Tuch DS, Makris N, et al. White matter abnormalities in dystonia normalize after botulinum toxin treatment. Neuroreport 2006;17(12):1251–5, ISSN: 09594965.

29. Egger K, Mueller J, Schocke M, et al. Voxel based morphometry reveals specific gray matter changes in primary dystonia. Mov Disord 2007;22(11): 1538–42, ISSN: 08853185.

30. Garraux G, Bauer A, Hanakawa T, et al. Changes in brain anatomy in focal hand dystonia. Ann Neurol 2004;55(5):736–9, ISSN: 03645134.

31. Dresel C, Haslinger B, Castrop F, et al. Silent event-related fMRI reveals deficient motor and enhanced somatosensory activation in orofacial dystonia. Brain 2006;129:36–46 [Epub 2005 Nov 9].

32. Blood AJ, Flaherty AW, Choi JK, et al. Basal ganglia activity remains elevated after movement in focal hand dystonia. Ann Neurol 2004;55(5):744–8.

33. Pujol J, Roset-Llobet J, Rosines-Cubells D, et al. Brain cortical activation during guitar-induced hand dystonia studied by functional MRI. Neuroimage 2000;12(3):257–67.

34. Toma K, Nakai T. Functional MRI in human motor control studies and clinical applications. Magn Reson Med Sci 2002;1(2):109–20.

35. Bucher SF, Seelos KC, Dodel RC, et al. Activation mapping in essential tremor with functional magnetic resonance imaging. Ann Neurol 1997; 41(1):32–40.

36. Berg D, Preibisch C, Hofmann E, et al. Cerebral activation pattern in primary writing tremor. J Neurol Neurosurg Psychiatr 2000;69(6):780–6.

37. Clark VP, Lai S, Deckel AW. Altered functional MRI responses in Huntington's disease. Neuroreport 2002;13(5):703–6.

38. Georgiou-Karistianis N, Sritharan A, Farrow M, et al. Increased cortical recruitment in Huntington's disease using a Simon task. Neuropsychologia 2007;45(8):1791–800 [Epub 2007 Jan 18].

39. Aron AR, Schlaghecken F, Fletcher PC, et al. Inhibition of subliminally primed responses is mediated by the caudate and thalamus: evidence from functional MRI and Huntington's disease. Brain 2003;126:713–23.

40. Thiruvady DR, Georgiou-Karistianis N, Egan GF, et al. Functional connectivity of the prefrontal cortex in Huntington's disease. J Neurol Neurosurg Psychiatr 2007;78(2):127–33 [Epub 2006 Oct 6].

41. Gavazzi C, Nave RD, Petralli R, et al. Combining functional and structural brain magnetic resonance imaging in Huntington disease. J Comput Assist Tomogr 2007;31(4):574–80.

42. Kim JS, Reading SA, Brashers-Krug T, et al. Functional MRI study of a serial reaction time task in Huntington's disease. Psychiatry Res 2004;131(1):23–30.

43. Hennenlotter A, Schroeder U, Erhard P, et al. Neural correlates associated with impaired disgust processing in pre-symptomatic Huntington's disease. Brain 2004;127:1446–53 [Epub 2004 Apr 16].

44. Zimbelman JL, Paulsen JS, Mikos A, et al. fMRI detection of early neural dysfunction in preclinical Huntington's disease. J Int Neuropsychol Soc 2007;13(5):758–69.

How Can Neuroimaging Help in the Diagnosis of Movement Disorders?

Helen Ling, BMBS, MSc, Andrew J. Lees, MD, FRCP, FMedSci*

KEYWORDS

- Movement disorders • Neuroimaging • MCP sign
- Eye-of-the-tiger sign • Pulvinar sign
- Hot-cross bun sign • Hummingbird sign
- Face-of-the-giant panda sign

The main role of computed axial tomography in the field of movement disorders was to exclude very uncommon but potentially reversible structural abnormalities including tumors, chronic subdural hematoma, and communicating hydrocephalus presenting with parkinsonism. In the past 20 years, magnetic resonance has had a far greater impact in facilitating accurate diagnosis but it would be fair to say that its clinical usefulness is much less than in some other neurologic fields such as cerebrovascular disease and multiple sclerosis. Dopamine transporter single-photon emission computed tomography (SPECT) imaging (DAT scan) on the other hand has proved to be a very helpful investigation in distinguishing benign tremulous Parkinson disease (PD) from atypical tremor syndromes and in a number of other clinical scenarios where the demonstration of nigrostriatal dopamine denervation is helpful.

In this article, we use eight case vignettes to illustrate how MR imaging findings can assist in the diagnosis of movement disorders and, in some cases, change the course of patient management.

CASE 1: A 68-YEAR-OLD MAN WITH TREMOR, ATAXIA, AND PARKINSONISM

A 68-year-old man developed postural tremor of his right hand at the age of 60. Two years later, his gait became progressively unsteady. There was no family history of relevance. Examination revealed a mild dysexecutive syndrome, bilateral Holmes tremors, a wide-based ataxic gait and symmetric bradykinesia. There was no response to L-dopa and an MR scan was ordered.

Neuroimaging

This patient had Holmes tremor, cerebellar ataxia, parkinsonism, and subtle cognitive dysfunction. At initial presentation he was thought to have tremulous PD. Coexisting cerebellar ataxia should also lead to consideration of atypical parkinsonian syndrome such as the cerebellar subtype of multiple system atrophy (MSA-C) or other inherited cerebellar ataxias such as spinocerebellar ataxia (SCA) type 2 and 3.

The MR imaging scan revealed increased T2 signal in the white matter of middle cerebellar peduncles (the "MCP sign") (Fig. 1). This is a characteristic feature observed in Fragile X tremor ataxia syndrome (FXTAS).[1] This is a recently recognized adult disorder that occurs in individuals who are carriers of premutation alleles (55–200 CGG repeats) of the Fragile X Mental Retardation (FMR1) gene, leading to production of toxic FMR1 mRNA and formation of ubiquitin-positive intranuclear inclusions in the neurons and astrocytes throughout the brain.

Prevalence of FXTAS is estimated at 1 in 8000 males older than 50 years in the general population and is still frequently unrecognized.[2] Presenting symptoms include postural or intention tremor

Reta Lila Weston Institute of Neurological Studies, Institute of Neurology, University College London, 1 Wakefield Street, London, WC1N 1PJ, UK
* Corresponding author.
E-mail address: alees@ion.ucl.ac.uk (A.J. Lees).

Neuroimag Clin N Am 20 (2010) 111–123
doi:10.1016/j.nic.2009.08.004

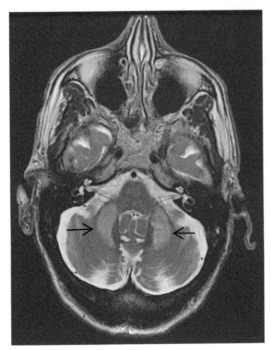

Fig. 1. Axial T2-weighted MR imaging demonstrates prominent increased signal intensity in the middle cerebellar peduncles, known as the "MCP sign" and moderate generalized cerebral atrophy.

The "MCP sign" can also be rarely observed in other conditions such as MSA-C, SCA type 6, Wilson disease, acquired hepatocerebral degeneration, cerebrovascular infarction, and dysplastic changes in neurofibromatosis.[7–12]

Other radiological findings observed in FXTAS include moderate to severe generalized brain atrophy and increased signal in T2-weighted images in periventricular and deep white matter of the cerebral hemispheres and corpus callosum.[1]

CASE 2: A 14-YEAR-OLD TEENAGER WITH PROGRESSIVE COGNITIVE DECLINE, DYSARTHRIA, DYSTONIA, AND SPASTIC GAIT

A 14-year-old boy presented with a 2-year history of progressive dysarthria, dystonia of upper limbs, and gait difficulty. His test results from school had declined markedly over the past year and he had personality change with frequent violent outbursts. He was an only child and had no family history of neurologic disorder. Examination showed bradyphrenia, dysarthria with palilalia, moderate limb dystonia and rigidity pyramidal signs, and a spastic gait.

Neuroimaging

In a young patient presenting with a mixed movement disorder, pyramidal abnormalities, and cognitive decline, the diagnosis of Wilson disease should always be ruled out. Rare neurodegenerative and neurometabolic disorders such as neuronal ceroid lipofuscinosis (Kuf disease), Westphal variant of Huntington disease (HD), neurodegeneration with brain iron accumulation (Hallervorden-Spatz syndrome), hexosaminidase A, or GM1 galactosidase deficiency should also be considered.

In this case, the finding of an "eye of the tiger" sign on neuroimaging led to the correct diagnosis of neurodegeneration with brain iron accumulation (Hallervorden-Spatz syndrome) (Fig. 2).

Neurodegeneration with brain iron accumulation (NBIA) is an autosomal recessive disorder characterized by dystonia, parkinsonism, and iron accumulation in the brain. Many patients with NBIA have mutations in the pantothenate kinase-2 gene (PANK-2) on chromosome 20p13.[13] The characteristic "eye of the tiger sign," with hyperintense signal changes in the central part of the globus pallidus representing iron deposition, is strongly correlated with PANK-2 mutation, and all PANK-2 mutation-positive patients are said to eventually exhibit this radiological finding.[14] Despite a recent case report describing the

followed by gait ataxia. Other common features include L-dopa unresponsive parkinsonism, frontal lobe signs leading to cognitive dysfunction, dysautonomia, and peripheral neuropathy. The disorder is more slowly progressive than MSA-C. A study showed that the frequency of FMR1 premutation alleles was 4 (2.4%) in 167 patients who received a clinical diagnosis of probable MSA-C.[3] Relevant family history includes children or grandchildren with mental retardation or behavioral disorders, female relatives with infertility, premature menopause, or family members with ataxia, psychiatric problems, dementia, or diagnosis of PD with dementia or multiple sclerosis.

The presence of the characteristic "MCP sign" with the finding of 87 CGG repeats (55–200) in the FMR1 gene led directly to the correct diagnosis in this case. The "MCP sign" is seen in 60% of males[4] and 13% of females[5] with the FXTAS permutation, so has limited sensitivity. Patients with both tremor and ataxia and who tested positive for the premutation but lack the "MCP sign" are diagnosed as having "probable" FXTAS. At autopsy, only a mild degree of spongiosis with occasional swollen axons are found in the MCP region despite the significantly abnormal appearance on MR imaging.[6]

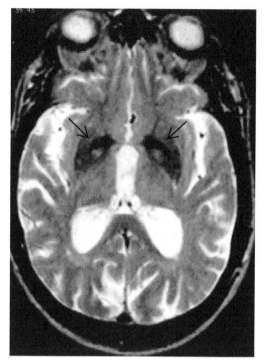

Fig. 2. Axial T2-weighted MR imaging demonstrates bilateral areas of hyperintensity within a region of hypointensity in the medial globus pallidus, also known as the "eye of the tiger sign."

disappearance of the "eye of the tiger" in a case with genetically confirmed PANK-2 mutation,[15] the sensitivity of this sign still approaches 100%. The reverse is also true, in that the "eye of the tiger" pattern is not observed in the MR imaging of PANK-2-negative patients.[14] Although NBIA with PANK-2 mutation is most commonly a disorder of childhood, there are some cases with juvenile or adult presentations with dystonia, parkinsonism, and pyramidal signs.[16] Severe dysarthria is often a prominent early finding.[16]

"Eye of the tiger" sign is not pathognomonic, as it has been reported in some parkinsonian syndromes including three patients with progressive supranuclear palsy (PSP),[17] one of whom was pathologically proven, one patient with early-onset levodopa-responsive parkinsonism,[18] and one patient with clinical diagnosis of corticobasal degeneration (CBD).[19] The clinical picture and age of onset is different in these disorders and should not lead to diagnostic confusion. On the other hand, the "eye of the tiger" sign has recently been reported in two cases of neuroferritinopathy, which is another NBIA condition of autosomal dominant inheritance that can closely resemble neurodegeneration with brain iron accumulation with the PANK-2 mutation.[20]

CASE 3: A 42-YEAR-OLD MAN WITH PROGRESSIVE COGNITIVE DECLINE, OROLINGUAL DYSKINESIA, PALATAL TREMOR, AND DYSTONIA OF THE LEGS

A 42-year-old man developed stereotyped hyperkinetic movements of the tongue and lips and slurred speech at the age of 35. His father and paternal grandmother had both developed a similar movement disorder in middle age. Examination revealed impairment of abstract reasoning, a dysexecutive syndrome, and the presence of some frontal release signs. Eye movements were abnormal with hypometric saccades and the use of head thrusts to initiate saccades. He had a slurring dysarthria, orofacial dyskinesia, and involuntary pouting with occasional facial grimacing. Palatal tremor at a frequency of 1 Hz was noted but ear clicking was not a feature. Lower limb examination revealed both dystonia and chorea of the right leg and a striatal right toe.

The following test results were normal or negative: full blood count, peripheral blood smear, copper studies, creatine kinase (CK), liver function test, nerve conduction studies, and genetic testing for Huntington disease.

Neuroimaging

The clinical picture and family history suggestive of an autosomal disorder raised the possibility of Huntington disease. The prominence of orofacial dyskinesias and the presence of both chorea and dystonia also raised the possibility of neuroacanthocytosis and McLeod syndrome. However, the absence of peripheral neuropathy on nerve conduction studies and a normal CK effectively excluded these disorders. Genetic test for Huntington disease was negative, ruling out Huntington disease. Some of the autosomally inherited spinocerebellar ataxias and ataxia telangiectasia and dentatorubropallidoluysian atrophy (DRPLA) may present with a movement disorder and cognitive deficit but cerebellar ataxia is usually prominent. Genetic testing for SCA 1 to 3, 6, and 7 DRPLA was negative in this case and ataxia telangiectasia was also ruled out by normal alpha fetoprotein levels.

Hypointense signal on T2-weighted MR imaging in the globus pallidus observed in this case raised the possibility of a neurodegenerative disorder in which brain iron accumulation was prominent (**Fig. 3**).[20] This is a characteristic feature in pantothenate kinase-associated neurodegeneration (Hallervorden-Spatz disease), infantile neuroaxonal dystrophy (INAD) with PLA mutation, aceruloplasminemia, and neuroferritinopathy. The clinical picture and radiological findings in this

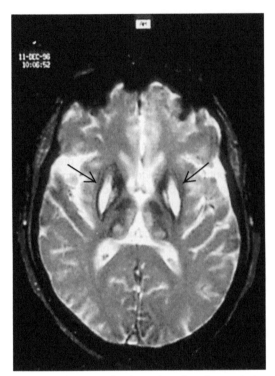

Fig. 3. Axial T2-weighted MR imaging demonstrates hyperintensity with surrounding hypointense cavitations affecting the putamen, pallidum, and thalamus.

case pointed more toward neuroferritinopathy or aceruloplasminemia, where more frequent involvements of the dentate and putamen are found radiologically and at postmortem and where the "eye of the tiger" sign is absent. Genetic testing confirmed the clinical suspicion of neuroferritinopathy in this case.

Neuroferritinopathy is an autosomal dominant condition that was first described in 2001[21] in families originating in the Cumbrian Lake District region of northwest England. A French family with neuroferritinopathy with the same mutation as the British family was later described.[22] Patients have a single adenine insertion between nucleotides 460 and 461 in exon 4 of the ferritin light chain gene.[21] Ferritin is an iron-storage protein and alteration of its structure by gene mutation leads to accumulation of extracellular iron in the brain, particularly in the basal ganglia. Excessive iron accumulation is toxic to the neurons, which leads to oxidative stress and neurodegeneration. The clinical suspicion of this disorder can be confirmed by the finding of serum ferritin being abnormally low or at the low end of the normal range. Definitive diagnosis is made by genetic testing confirming ferritin light chain gene mutation.

Patients present in their 20s to 40s with abnormal movements composed of dystonia, dysarthria, blepharospasm, chorea, spasticity, rigidity, and cognitive impairment of frontal subcortical dysfunction and sometimes the disease can progress rather acutely. These abnormal movements are characteristically asymmetric at initial presentation and remain asymmetrical despite gradual generalized involvement as the disease progresses. Predilection of the facial and buccolingual regions are common. Palatal tremor has been reported.[23] It is thought to be caused by iron deposition in the dentate nuclei, which is a component of the "Mollaret triangle" in addition to the inferior olivary and red nuclei.

A confluent area of hyperintensity involving globus pallidus and putamen with a rim of peripheral hypointensity is characteristic on MR imaging. This finding corresponds to the autopsy finding of cystic degeneration of the putamen and globus pallidus with fluid accumulation within the cysts.

In patients with palatal tremor, the MR imaging finding of inferior olivary nucleus hypertrophy suggests "symptomatic palatal tremor," and clinically, as in this case, is not associated with ear clicking. Symptomatic palatal tremor has also been reported in MSA, PSP, and late-onset Alexander disease where atrophy of the medulla oblongata in the presence of white matter lesions are helpful radiological findings.[24]

CASE 4: A 42-YEAR-OLD DRUG ADDICT WITH PARKINSONISM, EARLY GAIT INSTABILITY, AND FALLS BACKWARD

A 42-year-old Ukrainian man presented with progressive slurred speech, asymmetrical akinetic rigidity, gait difficulty, and emotional lability. He had a history of intravenous drug abuse. Examination revealed incontinent laughter, risus sardonicus, hypomimia, apraxia of eyelid opening, hypophonia, asymmetrical bradykinesia, and rigidity. He fell backward spontaneously and had a characteristic "cock walk gait" with an erect posture. His eye movements were normal. The symptoms did not improve with L-dopa therapy.

Neuroimaging

This middle-aged man developed a progressive parkinsonian syndrome with several features that would be unusual for PD such as gait difficulty falls backward, retropulsion, pseudobulbar symptoms, apraxia of eyelid opening, and poor L-dopa response within the first 2 years of illness. These symptoms more closely resemble PSP[25] with the exception of a "cock walk gait," in which patients walk on their toes with elbows flexed and an erect trunk. The clinical picture also resembled chronic manganism seen in miners exposed to ore fumes.[26] His history of drug abuse and his country of origin raised the possibility of "ephedrone" abuse. This new form of manganese poisoning has been reported in drug addicts in Russia, Ukraine, Georgia, and Estonia who intravenously inject themselves with a cocktail of pseudoephedrine (cold remedy bought over the counter), mixed with potassium permanganate and vinegar as oxidants to produce methcathinone, a central nervous stimulant structurally similar to methamphetamine.[27]

The clinical syndrome of "ephedrone" toxicity is similar to the original reports of chronic manganism observed in Chilean miners following inhalation of ore dust.[28] Other common causes of manganese poisoning can be seen in workers in alloy plant or dry battery factories, exposure to manganese-containing pesticides, prolonged total parenteral nutrition, and chronic liver disease with resulting impaired hepatic manganese metabolism.

In this case, the symmetric hyperintense T1-weighted signal in the globus pallidus was suggestive of deposition of paramagnetic substance such as manganese, iron, and copper (Fig. 4).[29] This characteristic MR imaging finding helped confirm the clinical suspicion manganese poisoning from "ephedrone" abuse. Increased signal on T1-weighted MR imaging can be caused by other conditions including accumulation of fat, melanin, calcifications, hemorrhages, and hypoxic conditions such as carbon monoxide poisoning, nonketotic hyperglycemia, and neurofibromatosis.

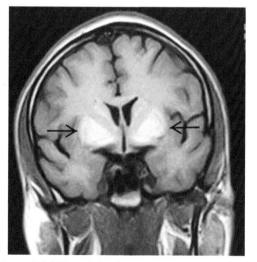

Fig. 4. Axial T1-weighted MR imaging demonstrates marked hyperintensity in the medial and lateral part of globus pallidus and to lesser degree in the putamen outlined by a hyperintense rim.

In "manganic encephalopathy," brain regions commonly involved include globus pallidus, particularly in the medial region, substantia nigra, subthalamic nucleus and lateral putamen.[27] Involvement of the dentate nucleus can also occur. The extent of hyperintensity on T1-weighted MR imaging is thought to correlate with the concentration of manganese in the body; thus the closer the proximity to "ephedrone" exposure, the more intense and widespread the abnormal T1 hyperintensity signal changes are observed. In patients who have stopped using "ephedrone" for more than a year, their MR imaging improves even when residual neurologic impairment is seen.[30] Delayed progression of extrapyramidal symptoms despite removal from manganese exposure has also been reported in some individuals. Dopamine transporter SPECT 123I-Ioflupane (DaTSCAN) imaging is normal in these patients, supporting a post-synaptic "supranigral" cause of parkinsonism.[27] In contrast to MPTP toxicity, which also occurs in drug addicts,[31] individuals with "ephedronic encephalopathy" are nonresponsive to L-dopa.

Clinical suspicion can also be supported by the high concentration of manganese level measured in the blood or in pubic hair samples (>1.1 μg/g), even after prolonged cessation of "ephedrone exposure" of more than 1 year.[27]

CASE 5: A 22-YEAR-OLD WOMAN WITH RAPIDLY PROGRESSIVE COGNITIVE IMPAIRMENT AND CEREBELLAR ATAXIA

A 22-year-old university student presented with a 4-month history of profound behavioral changes and psychotic behavior. She then complained of persistent painful dysesthesia in the hands and feet and unsteady gait and cognitive decline were apparent. She had no previous medical history or family history of any neurologic disorder. Examination revealed Mini-Mental State Exam score of 22/30, intermittent myoclonus of the limbs, an intention tremor of both hands, and a wide-based ataxic gait.

Neuroimaging

This young woman had an initial psychiatric presentation followed by rapidly progressive dementia with cerebellar ataxia and myoclonus. The differential diagnoses included toxic infectious, paraneoplastic, or autoimmune causes; brain tumor or lymphoma; or rare mitochondrial encephalopathy. The rapid progression also raised the possibility of new variant Creutzfeldt-Jakob Disease (vCJD).[32]

MR imaging is an important diagnostic tool for CJD and can help differentiate sporadic (sCJD) and variant subtypes (Fig. 5). The "pulvinar sign" is the characteristic radiological finding of vCJD with symmetric hyperintense signal on T2-weighted MR imaging within the pulvinar region of the thalamus.[33] It has a sensitivity of over 70% and a specificity of almost 100% for vCJD and can be seen on T2-weighted image as well as proton-density–weighted, fluid attenuation inversion recovery (FLAIR), and diffusion-weighted images.[34] FLAIR images have the highest sensitivity among other sequences. This radiological feature is incorporated in the operational diagnostic criteria for vCJD.[35] Another finding is high T2 signal in the mediodorsal thalamic nucleus and can be seen in about half of vCJD cases, thus is less specific. The combination of "pulvinar sign" and hyperintense signal in the mediodorsal thalamic nucleus is sometimes referred to as the "hockey-stick sign" on axial scans.[36] T1-signal change or contrast enhancement is not observed in vCJD.[34] High T2-signal change in the pulvinar has also been reported in sCJD.[37] The maximal hyperintense signal changes in the reported case, however, were in the caudate head and putamen bilaterally, and would not therefore have fulfilled the World Health Organization's revised definition of the "pulvinar sign," defined as "bilateral symmetric pulvinar high signal relative to the signal intensity of other deep gray matter nuclei and cortical gray matter."[38]

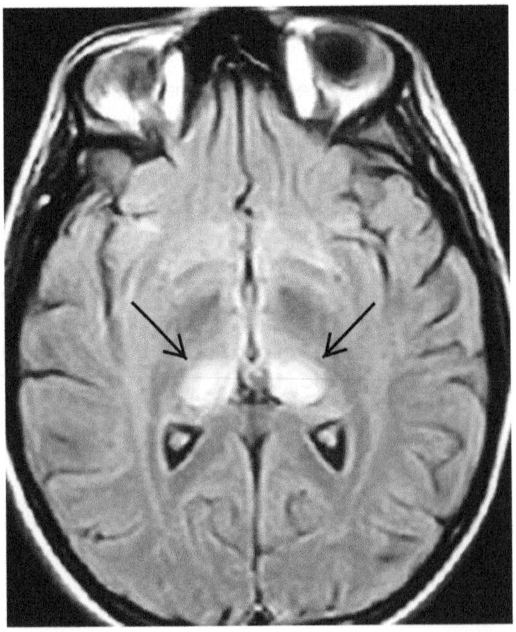

"Pulvinar sign" has been reported in rare cases of postinfectious encephalitis, cat-scratch disease, intracranial hypertension, and Alpers syndrome (progressive infantile poliodystrophy, a rare mitochondrial encephalomyelopathy).[36] However, the clinical picture of these disorders does not resemble vCJD and should not lead to diagnostic confusion.

In patients clinically suspected to have vCJD, a clinical diagnosis can be made by assessing the clinical features, characteristic MR imaging findings, serial EEGs, cerebrospinal fluid (CSF) study for 14-3-3 protein, positive tonsil biopsy, and genetic testing for methionine homozygous at codon 129. An accurate and early clinical diagnosis is important to exclude other treatable disorders and to avoid invasive brain biopsy. In vCJD, EEG shows nonspecific generalized slowing, in contrast to the typical appearance of periodic sharp wave complexes seen in sCJD.[35] The 14-3-3 protein from CSF study is detected in 50% to 60% of vCJD cases with a specificity of up to 94%; whereas the sensitivity and specificity of positive 14-3-3 protein for sCJD are 96% and 74% respectively.[35] In vCJD the pathologic prion protein also infects the peripheral lymphoid tissue including the tonsils, so positive tonsil biopsy can allow positive confirmation of the diagnosis. All cases of vCJD are homozygous for methionine at codon 129 in prion protein gene analysis.[35]

CASE 6: A 54-YEAR-OLD MAN WITH PROGRESSIVE ATAXIA, FOLLOWED BY PARKINSONISM, OROFACIAL DYSKINESIA, AND DYSAUTONOMIA

A 54-year-old engineer developed erectile dysfunction followed a year later by progressive clumsiness and slurred speech. Over the following year, he became increasingly unsteady on his feet and frequently spilled drinks because of clumsiness of his hands. Over the next 2 years his movements became slow and he complained of stiffness and light headedness and episodes of urinary retention required self-catheterization. His motor symptoms transiently and partially improved with L-dopa but he experienced orofacial dystonia while taking the medication. There was no relevant family history and he never drank alcohol excessively. Examination revealed normal cognition, jerky pursuit and dysmetric saccadic eye movements, anterocollis, orofacial dystonia, and truncal ataxia. Routine blood tests, thyroid function tests, vitamin E level, autoantibodies screen, and genetic tests for

Fig. 5. Axial T2-weighted MR imaging demonstrates symmetric high signal intensity in the pulvinar region of the thalamic nucleus, also known as the "pulvinar sign."

SCA 1 to 3, 6, and 7 and Friedreich ataxia were either normal or negative. Autonomic function test showed marked cardiovascular autonomic failure with orthostatic hypotension.

Neuroimaging

This patient presented with atypical parkinsonism with early autonomic dysfunction and cerebellar signs. This is the classical presentation of MSA that usually manifests in middle age and progresses relentlessly with a mean survival of 6 to 9 years.[39] Initial L-dopa response occurs in a third of patients, however 90% of them are unresponsive on long-term follow-up. Orofacial dystonia is a feature observed in more than half of all MSA patients and may occur spontaneously or more usually as a complication of L-dopa therapy. Disproportionate anterocollis is another characteristic feature seen in MSA. Early urinary incontinence and syncope are characteristic for MSA and contrast with the later autonomic involvement often seen in Parkinson disease (PD). Early erectile dysfunction is also common and urinary retention as occurred in this case can rarely be an early symptom. There are two subtypes of MSA: parkinsonian (MSA-P) and cerebellar (MSA-C) subtypes. Neuropathologically, all subtypes of MSA are collectively characterized by the finding of α-synuclein glial cytoplasmic inclusions in the striatum and cerebellum (GCIs).[40]

The clinical differential diagnoses for this patient would include the following: other atypical parkinsonian syndromes, adult-onset cerebellar ataxia that can be hereditary despite a negative family history (eg, Friedreich ataxia), SCA, FXTA syndrome, and autoimmune conditions in association with Anti-GAD in celiac disease, anti-Yo and anti-Hu in paraneoplastic syndromes. Toxic and metabolic conditions (eg, hypothyroidism, alcohol-related cerebellar degeneration) should also be considered, as some of these are potentially reversible.

Neuroimaging is not included in the consensus diagnostic criteria of MSA.[41] Nevertheless, typical neurologic findings can assist in differentiating MSA from other causes of parkinsonism and cerebellar ataixia (Fig. 6).[42] The "hot-cross bun" sign observed in this case is characterized by cruciform signal hyperintensity on T2-weighted images in mid pons, which resembles a hot-cross bun, traditionally baked on the last Thursday before Easter (see Fig. 6A).[43] This finding is thought to correspond to the loss of pontine neurons and myelinated transverse cerebellar fibers with preservation of the corticospinal tracts. However, this sign is not specific to MSA and has been reported in other conditions such as SCA. The more common typical radiological findings in MSA include atrophy of the cerebellum, most prominently in the vermis, middle cerebellar peduncles, pons, and lower brainstem. In addition to putaminal atrophy, a characteristic hypointense signal in T2 with hyperintense rim, corresponding to reactive gliosis and astrogliosis, can be

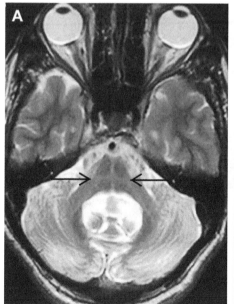
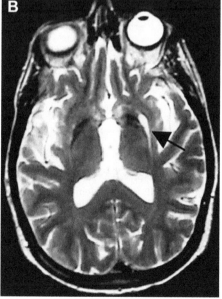

Fig. 6. (A) Axial T2-weighted MR imaging demonstrates cruciform hyperintense signal changes in mid pons, the so-called "hot-cross bun sign." (B) Axial T2-weighted MR imaging demonstrates hypointensity in association with hyperintense rim in the external putamen, which is termed "slit-like void sign."

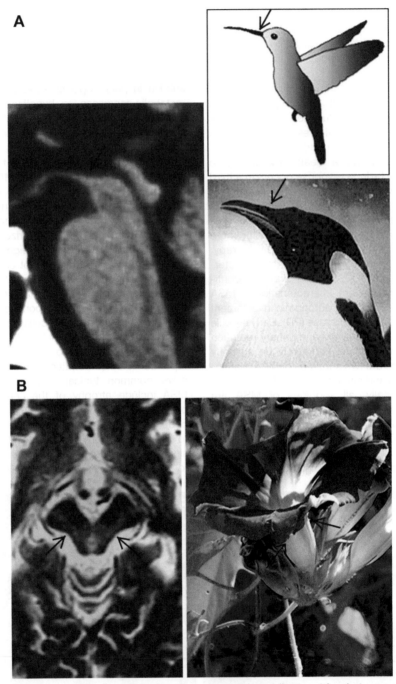

Fig. 7. (*A*) Sagittal T1-MR imaging demonstrates volume loss in the midbrain with relative preservation of the pons. The midbrain tegmentum has lost its normal convexity giving it the appearance of a hummingbird (or penguin), also known as the "hummingbird sign." (*B*) T2-weighted axial MR imaging demonstrates "Mickey mouse" or "morning glory" sign with concavity of the lateral margin of midbrain tegmentum.

observed in the external putamen, and is termed "slit-like void sign" (see **Fig. 6**B).[44,45] This combination of hypointense and hyperintense putaminal signal change is specific for MSA and its finding can be used to differentiate MSA from PSP and PD.[45] Hypointensity alone without hyperintense rim is a sensitive radiological feature but nonspecific for MSA.[45]

CASE 7: A 71-YEAR-OLD MAN WITH GAIT DIFFICULTY, FREQUENT FALLS, AKINETIC RIGIDITY, AND HYPOPHONIC SPEECH

A 71-year-old retired painter presented with 2-year history of increasing difficulty with initiation of gait. He had frequent falls with a tendency to topple backward. He developed a soft growling speech, apraxia of eyelid opening, and symmetric bradykinesia. He sometimes cried inappropriately but his cognitive function was otherwise thought to be normal. He had no family history of neurologic disorder.

Examination revealed positive applause sign, utilization behavior, and a positive bilateral grasp and palmomental reflex, a staring appearance with reduced blinking, apraxia of eyelid opening, hypophonic dysarthria, supranuclear up and down gaze palsy, and axial rigidity. He walked with a broad-based shuffling gait and the pull test was positive. His symptoms did not improve with L-dopa treatment.

Neuroimaging

This elderly man had an atypical parkinsonian syndrome characterized by early postural instability and falls backward, a vertical supranuclear gaze palsy, axial rigidity, pseudobulbar palsy, frontal lobe signs, and a poor response to L-dopa. These are characteristic features of PSP, also known as Richardson disease. It has a prevalence of 5 per 100,000, but is commonly underdiagnosed. The clinical features are quite different from PD or other atypical parkinsonian syndromes such as MSA. However, there is a subgroup of PSP patients, known as PSP-Parkinsonism (PSP-P), which presents with asymmetrical bradykinesia, jerky tremor, and an initial L-dopa response without vertical gaze palsy. Other unusual presenting features of PSP include primary gait freezing, early frontotemporal dementia, and corticobasal syndrome.

MR imaging of the brain can be normal in the early stages of disease. Nevertheless, certain MR imaging features can greatly assist in making the diagnosis especially in patients with PSP-P or an atypical presentation (Fig. 7). The first radiological clue for PSP would be the presence of striking hyperextension of the neck on sagittal MR imaging. The characteristic MR imaging feature is selective atrophy of the midbrain in association with preservation of the pons. The resulting atrophy of the midbrain tegmentum gives a distinctive concavity with the appearance of the beak of a hummingbird or king penguin, and is termed the "hummingbird"[46] or "penguin" sign (see Fig. 7A).[47] Quantitative measurements of midbrain atrophy have been shown to improve diagnostic accuracy of PSP. Midbrain diameter in PSP (13.4 mm) was shown to be significantly lower than that of PD (18.5 mm).[48] Recent study indicated that the surface area of midbrain of PSP (56 mm^2) was significantly smaller than that

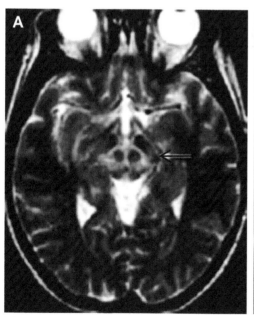
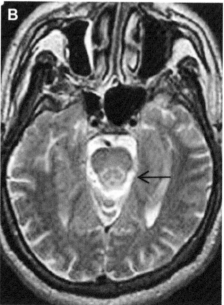

Fig. 8. (*A*) Axial T2-weighted MR imaging demonstrates "face of the giant panda sign" with hyperintensity in the midbrain tegmentum with relative sparing of the red nuclei, part of the pars reticulate of the substantia nigra and superior colliculus. (*B*) Axial T2-weighted MR imaging demonstrates "face of the miniature panda sign" within the pontine tegmentum with similar hyperintense signal changes as seen in the midbrain tegmentum.

Table 1
Useful characteristic MR imaging findings to assist in diagnosing movement disorders

Movement Disorder	Characteristic Signs on MR Imaging
Fragile X tremor ataxia syndrome (FXTA)	"MCP sign" with prominent increased T2 signal intensity in the middle cerebellar peduncles
Pantothenate kinase-associated neurodegeneration (PKAN) (Hallervorden-Spatz syndrome)	"Eye of the tiger sign" with bilateral areas of hyperintensity within a region of hypointensity in the medial globus pallidus in T2-weighted images
Neuroferritinopathy	Hyperintensity with surrounding hypointense cavitations affecting the putamen, pallidum, and thalamus in T2-weighted images
Manganese toxicity	Hyperintensity in globus pallidus and putamen outlined by a hyperintense rim in T1-weighted images
Variant Creutzfeldt-Jakob disease (vCJD)	"Pulvinar sign" with symmetric hyperintensity in the pulvinar region of the thalamic nucleus in T2-weighted images
Multiple system atrophy (MSA)	"Hot-cross bun sign" with cruciform hyperintensity in mid pons in T2-weighted images, and "slit-like void sign" with hypointensity in association with hyperintense rim in the external putamen in T2-weighted images
Progressive supranuclear palsy (PSP)	"Hummingbird" or "penguin" sign with volume loss in the midbrain and relative preservation of the pons in sagittal T1-weighted images, and "Mickey mouse" or "morning glory" sign with concavity of the lateral margin of midbrain tegmentum on T2-weighted axial images
Wilson disease	"Face of the giant panda sign" with hyperintensity in the midbrain tegmentum with sparing of the red nuclei, substantia nigra and superior colliculus in T2-weighted images, and "face of the miniature panda sign" with similar appearance within the pontine tegmentum

of MSA-P (97.2 mm^2), PD (103 mm^2), and healthy controls (117 mm^2). Some overlaps of the area measurements were observed in PSP and MSA-P, but the ratio of the area of the midbrain to pons was significantly smaller in PSP when compared with MSA-P.[47]

On axial views, the selective atrophy of the midbrain tegmentum with relative preservation of the tectum and cerebral peduncles produces the "Mickey mouse" sign (see **Fig. 7**B). Sometimes, the concavity of the lateral margin of the midbrain tegmentum is referred to as the "morning glory" sign and has high specificity but rather low sensitivity for PSP.

Other radiological findings of PSP include dilatation of the third ventricle, particularly the posterior portion, signal change in the periaqueductal gray matter indicative of gliosis, and atrophy of the superior cerebellar peduncle, which has a specificity of 94% and sensitivity of 74% and can aid the differentiation of PSP from MSA-P and PD.[49] "Eye of the tiger" sign with hypointensity signal change in T2, a common finding in pantothenate kinase-associated neurodegeneration (PKAN), can occasionally be observed in PSP, indicating the presence of iron deposition in the putamen.[17]

CASE 8: A 24-YEAR-OLD WOMAN WITH PROGRESSIVE BILATERAL ACTION TREMOR, JAW-OPENING DYSTONIA, AND DYSARTHRIA FOR 1 YEAR

A 24-year-old student nurse presented with a 1-year history of progressive bilateral action tremor of both hands. A few months later, her speech became slurred and her intellectual capacity declined and a friend commented that she had become more irritable and irascible. Her younger brother had died of liver failure at the age of 11. Examination revealed facial grimacing, jaw-opening dystonia, drooling, spastic dysarthria, postural and wing-beating tremor, and bilateral rigidity. A Kayser-Fleischer (KF) ring was noted on slit lamp examination.

Neuroimaging

This patient had a mixture of abnormal movements including orofacial dystonia, parkinsonism, and action tremor as well as cognitive impairment. Differential diagnoses included the Westphal variant of HD, PKAN, SCA2 and 3, neuroacanthocytosis, and Wilson disease. The characteristic KF ring, which is composed of copper deposition within the Descement membrane of the cornea, is characteristic of Wilson disease and is seen in more than 98% of cases with neurologic presentation.[50] The patient's brother most likely died of hepatic presentation of Wilson disease.

Wilson disease is an autosomal recessive disorder that results from mutation within the copper-transporting ATP7B gene localized on chromosome 13, leading to progressive copper accumulation. Diagnosis of Wilson disease can be confirmed by the presence of a markedly reduced plasma ceruloplasmin level and excessive 24-hour urinary copper excretion of more than 100 μg. DNA analysis for ATP7B mutation can confirm the diagnosis of Wilson disease; however, the diversity of mutations in the ATP7B gene in Wilson disease limits the use of genetic testing for routine diagnosis.

Neuroimaging findings can assist in the diagnosis of Wilson disease in individuals with equivocal copper studies and where there is doubt about the presence of a K-F ring on clinical examination (**Fig. 8**). Abnormalities on MR imaging are always seen in symptomatic patients with neurologic presentation of Wilson disease.[51,52] Typical MR imaging appearances include hyperintense signal on T2-weighted images, sometimes with a central core of hypointensity and are seen consistently in the basal ganglia.[53] Other structures include cerebral white matter, and infratentorial structures are sometimes involved. A characteristic finding is "face of the giant panda" sign, which corresponds to hyperintensity signal change in T2-weighted images in the midbrain tegmentum with sparing of the red nuclei (eyes of the panda), lateral aspect of the pars reticulate of the substantia nigra (ears), and superior colliculus (mouth) (see **Fig. 8**A).[54] Occasionally, similar hyperintense signal changes can be observed in the pontine tegmentum, which is termed "face of the miniature panda" sign (see **Fig. 8**B). Several studies have shown positive correlations between the regions with radiological signal changes and clinical symptoms. With effective chelation treatment, abnormalities on MR imaging can disappear.[55]

SUMMARY

These eight case reports illustrate how MR imaging can be a valuable investigation in the diagnosis of movement disorders (**Table 1**). The radiological findings are never diagnostic in themselves, but, taken in the context of the clinical picture can point the way to the correct diagnosis. In some rare conditions such as FXTA syndrome and vCJD, the typical neuroimaging findings may be the first diagnostic clue and can avoid a battery of extensive and wasteful investigations.

It is likely that in the next few years, new neuroradiological MR techniques will have a far greater impact on the routine clinical practice of movement disorders.

REFERENCES

1. Brunberg JA, Jacquemont S, Hagerman RJ, et al. Fragile X premutation carriers: characteristic MR imaging findings of adult male patients with progressive cerebellar and cognitive dysfunction. AJNR Am J Neuroradiol 2002;23(10):1757–66.
2. Jacquemont S, Hagerman RJ, Leehey MA, et al. Penetrance of the fragile X-associated tremor/ataxia syndrome in a premutation carrier population. JAMA 2004;291(4):460–9.
3. Berry-Kravis E, Abrams L, Coffey SM, et al. Fragile X-associated tremor/ataxia syndrome: clinical features, genetics, and testing guidelines. Mov Disord 2007;22(14):2018–30, quiz 2140.
4. Cohen S, Masyn K, Adams J, et al. Molecular and imaging correlates of the fragile X-associated tremor/ataxia syndrome. Neurology 2006;67(8):1426–31.
5. Adams JS, Adams PE, Nguyen D, et al. Volumetric brain changes in females with fragile X-associated tremor/ataxia syndrome (FXTAS). Neurology 2007;69(9):851–9.
6. Greco CM, Berman RF, Martin RM, et al. Neuropathology of fragile X-associated tremor/ataxia syndrome (FXTAS). Brain 2006;129(Pt 1):243–55.
7. Schulz JB, Klockgether T, Petersen D, et al. Multiple system atrophy: natural history, MRI morphology, and dopamine receptor imaging with 123IBZM-SPECT. J Neurol Neurosurg Psychiatr 1994;57(9):1047–56.
8. Nakagawa N, Katayama T, Makita Y, et al. A case of spinocerebellar ataxia type 6 mimicking olivopontocerebellar atrophy. Neuroradiology 1999;41(7):501–3.
9. Matsuura T, Sasaki H, Tashiro K. Atypical MR findings in Wilson's disease: pronounced lesions in the dentate nucleus causing tremor. J Neurol Neurosurg Psychiatr 1998;64(2):161.
10. Lee J, Lacomis D, Comu S, et al. Acquired hepatocerebral degeneration: MR and pathologic findings. AJNR Am J Neuroradiol 1998;19(3):485–7.
11. Akiyama K, Takizawa S, Tokuoka K, et al. Bilateral middle cerebellar peduncle infarction caused by traumatic vertebral artery dissection. Neurology 2001;56(5):693–4.
12. Menor F, Marti-Bonmati L, Arana E, et al. Neurofibromatosis type 1 in children: MR imaging and follow-up studies of central nervous system findings. Eur J Radiol 1998;26(2):121–31.
13. Zhou B, Westaway SK, Levinson B, et al. A novel pantothenate kinase gene (PANK2) is defective in Hallervorden-Spatz syndrome. Nat Genet 2001;28(4):345–9.
14. Hayflick SJ, Hartman M, Coryell J, et al. Brain MRI in neurodegeneration with brain iron accumulation with and without PANK2 mutations. AJNR Am J Neuroradiol 2006;27(6):1230–3.
15. Kumar N, Boes CJ, Babovic-Vuksanovic D, et al. The "eye-of-the-tiger" sign is not pathognomonic of the PANK2 mutation. Arch Neurol 2006;63(2):292–3.
16. Hayflick SJ, Westaway SK, Levinson B, et al. Genetic, clinical, and radiographic delineation of Hallervorden-Spatz syndrome. N Engl J Med 2003;348(1):33–40.
17. Davie CA, Barker GJ, Machado C, et al. Proton magnetic resonance spectroscopy in Steele-Richardson-Olszewski syndrome. Mov Disord 1997;12(5):767–71.
18. Barbosa ER, Bittar MS, Bacheschi LA, et al. [Precocious Parkinson's disease associated with "eye-of-the-tiger" type pallidal lesions]. Arq Neuropsiquiatr 1995;53(2):294–7 [in Portuguese].
19. Molinuevo JL, Munoz E, Valldeoriola F, et al. The eye of the tiger sign in cortical-basal ganglionic degeneration. Mov Disord 1999;14(1):169–71.
20. McNeill A, Birchall D, Hayflick SJ, et al. T2* and FSE MRI distinguishes four subtypes of neurodegeneration with brain iron accumulation. Neurology 2008;70(18):1614–9.
21. Curtis AR, Fey C, Morris CM, et al. Mutation in the gene encoding ferritin light polypeptide causes dominant adult-onset basal ganglia disease. Nat Genet 2001;28(4):350–4.
22. Chinnery PF, Curtis AR, Fey C, et al. Neuroferritinopathy in a French family with late onset dominant dystonia. J Med Genet 2003;40(5):e69.
23. Wills AJ, Sawle GV, Guilbert PR, et al. Palatal tremor and cognitive decline in neuroferritinopathy. J Neurol Neurosurg Psychiatr 2002;73(1):91–2.
24. Kulkarni PK, Muthane UB, Taly AB, et al. Palatal tremor, progressive multiple cranial nerve palsies, and cerebellar ataxia: a case report and review of literature of palatal tremors in neurodegenerative disease. Mov Disord 1999;14(4):689–93.
25. Steele JC, Richardson JC, Olszewski J. Progressive supranuclear palsy. A heterogeneous degeneration involving the brain stem, basal ganglia and cerebellum with vertical gaze and pseudobulbar palsy, nuchal dystonia and dementia. Arch Neurol 1964;10:333–59.
26. Huang CC, Chu NS, Lu CS, et al. Cock gait in manganese intoxication. Mov Disord 1997;12(5):807–8.
27. Selikhova M, Fedoryshyn L, Matviyenko Y, et al. Parkinsonism and dystonia caused by the illicit use of ephedrone—a longitudinal study. Mov Disord 2008;23(15):2224–31.
28. Couper J. On the effects of black oxide of manganese when inhaled into the lungs. Br Ann Med Pharmacol 1837;1:41–2.
29. Lucchini R, Albini E, Placidi D, et al. Brain magnetic resonance imaging and manganese exposure. Neurotoxicology 2000;21(5):769–75.

30. Sanotsky Y, Lesyk R, Fedoryshyn L, et al. Manganic encephalopathy due to "ephedrone" abuse. Mov Disord 2007;22(9):1337–43.

31. Ballard PA, Tetrud JW, Langston JW. Permanent human parkinsonism due to 1-methyl-4-phenyl-1,2,3,6-tetrahydropyridine (MPTP): seven cases. Neurology 1985;35(7):949–56.

32. Zerr I, Schulz-Schaeffer WJ, Giese A, et al. Current clinical diagnosis in Creutzfeldt-Jakob disease: identification of uncommon variants. Ann Neurol 2000;48(3):323–9.

33. Zeidler M, Sellar RJ, Collie DA, et al. The pulvinar sign on magnetic resonance imaging in variant Creutzfeldt-Jakob disease. Lancet 2000;355(9213): 1412–8.

34. Collie DA, Summers DM, Sellar RJ, et al. Diagnosing variant Creutzfeldt-Jakob disease with the pulvinar sign: MR imaging findings in 86 neuropathologically confirmed cases. AJNR Am J Neuroradiol 2003; 24(8):1560–9.

35. Will RG, Zeidler M, Stewart GE, et al. Diagnosis of new variant Creutzfeldt-Jakob disease. Ann Neurol 2000;47(5):575–82.

36. Tschampa HJ, Zerr I, Urbach H. Radiological assessment of Creutzfeldt-Jakob disease. Eur Radiol 2007; 17(5):1200–11.

37. Tschampa HJ, Murtz P, Flacke S, et al. Thalamic involvement in sporadic Creutzfeldt-Jakob disease: a diffusion-weighted MR imaging study. AJNR Am J Neuroradiol 2003;24(5):908–15.

38. The revision of the surveillance case definition for variant Creutzfeldt-Jakob disease (vCJD): report of a WHO Consultation. Edinburgh, United Kingdom. WHO; 2001. Available at: http://www.who.int/emc.

39. Bhidayasiri R, Ling H. Multiple system atrophy. Neurologist 2008;14(4):224–37.

40. Papp MI, Kahn JE, Lantos PL. Glial cytoplasmic inclusions in the CNS of patients with multiple system atrophy (striatonigral degeneration, olivopontocerebellar atrophy and Shy-Drager syndrome). J Neurol Sci 1989;94(1–3):79–100.

41. Gilman S, Low PA, Quinn N, et al. Consensus statement on the diagnosis of multiple system atrophy. J Neurol Sci 1999;163(1):94–8.

42. Schrag A, Good CD, Miszkiel K, et al. Differentiation of a typical parkinsonian syndromes with routine MRI. Neurology 2000;54(3):697–702.

43. Schrag A, Kingsley D, Phatouros C, et al. Clinical usefulness of magnetic resonance imaging in multiple system atrophy. J Neurol Neurosurg Psychiatr 1998;65(1):65–71.

44. Lang AE, Curran T, Provias J, et al. Striatonigral degeneration: iron deposition in putamen correlates with the slit-like void signal of magnetic resonance imaging. Can J Neurol Sci 1994;21(4):311–8.

45. Kraft E, Schwarz J, Trenkwalder C, et al. The combination of hypointense and hyperintense signal changes on T2-weighted magnetic resonance imaging sequences: a specific marker of multiple system atrophy? Arch Neurol 1999;56(2): 225–8.

46. Kato N, Arai K, Hattori T. Study of the rostral midbrain atrophy in progressive supranuclear palsy. J Neurol Sci 2003;210(1–2):57–60.

47. Oba H, Yagishita A, Terada H, et al. New and reliable MRI diagnosis for progressive supranuclear palsy. Neurology 2005;64(12):2050–5.

48. Warmuth-Metz M, Naumann M, Csoti I, et al. Measurement of the midbrain diameter on routine magnetic resonance imaging: a simple and accurate method of differentiating between Parkinson disease and progressive supranuclear palsy. Arch Neurol 2001;58(7):1076–9.

49. Paviour DC, Price SL, Stevens JM, et al. Quantitative MRI measurement of superior cerebellar peduncle in progressive supranuclear palsy. Neurology 2005;64(4):675–9.

50. Ala A, Walker AP, Ashkan K, et al. Wilson's disease. Lancet 2007;369(9559):397–408.

51. Thuomas KA, Aquilonius SM, Bergstrom K, et al. Magnetic resonance imaging of the brain in Wilson's disease. Neuroradiology 1993;35(2):134–41.

52. Roh JK, Lee TG, Wie BA, et al. Initial and follow-up brain MRI findings and correlation with the clinical course in Wilson's disease. Neurology 1994;44(6): 1064–8.

53. Magalhaes AC, Caramelli P, Menezes JR, et al. Wilson's disease: MRI with clinical correlation. Neuroradiology 1994;36(2):97–100.

54. Hitoshi S, Iwata M, Yoshikawa K. Mid-brain pathology of Wilson's disease: MRI analysis of three cases. J Neurol Neurosurg Psychiatr 1991;54(7):624–6.

55. Stefano Zagami A, Boers PM. Disappearing "face of the giant panda". Neurology 2001;56(5):665.

The Role of Imaging in the Surgical Treatment of Movement Disorders

Ludvic Zrinzo, MD, MSc, FRCSEd (Neuro.Surg)[a,b,*]

KEYWORDS

- Imaging • MRI • Neurosurgery • Deep brain stimulation
- Movement disorders

FUNCTIONAL NEUROSURGERY

Functional neurosurgery involves precise surgical targeting of anatomic structures to modulate neurologic function. The ultimate aim is to improve the symptoms and quality of life of patients suffering from chronic neurologic disorders; this demands minimal risk of inflicting morbidity and mortality. Well-established indications for functional neurosurgery include movement disorders such as Parkinson disease (PD),[1,2] several forms of dystonia,[3,4] essential tremor,[5,6] and chronic pain.[7,8] Other indications proposed in recent literature, either novel or revisited, are less well established but hold promise for patients with chronic debilitating conditions including cluster headache,[9] Tourette syndrome,[10–12] obsessive compulsive disorder,[13–15] severe refractory depression,[16] and epilepsy.[17–19] This article focuses on the role of imaging in the surgical treatment of movement disorders.

Imaging has played a central role in the practice of functional neurosurgery since its inception. The current situation and likely future directions are best appreciated by reviewing their parallel development.

THE EARLY YEARS OF FUNCTIONAL NEUROSURGERY

Initial attempts to surgically control abnormal movements involved drastic measures. Functional neurosurgery originated in the late nineteenth century when Victor Horsley[20,21] extirpated large areas of motor cortex for the relief of athetosis. Desperate assaults on the pyramidal system, at cranial and spinal levels, were invariably accompanied by significant motor deficit.[22] Meyers[23,24] suggested the basal ganglia as a target for surgery for involuntary movement disorders in the following decades, and in the 1940s the target for ablation moved to the so-called extrapyramidal system. Although these adventurous, open procedures proved that effective surgery need not impose significant neurologic deficit, they were associated with prohibitive mortality rates.[23,25]

Cooper[26,27] refocused attention on the basal ganglia as a target for surgical interventions when he noted the beneficial effect on contralateral tremor after accidentally ligating the anterior choroidal artery (AChA) in a patient with PD. The variable vascular territory of the AChA makes this an inconsistent way of performing basal ganglia

Funding: This work was undertaken at UCL/UCLH and was partly funded by the Department of Health NIHR Biomedical Research Centres funding scheme. The Unit of Functional Neurosurgery, Queen Square, London is supported by the Parkinson's Appeal.
[a] Victor Horsley Department of Neurosurgery, National Hospital for Neurology and Neurosurgery, University College London Hospitals NHS Foundation Trust, Box 146, Second Floor, 33 Queen Square, London, WC1N 3BG, UK
[b] Unit of Functional Neurosurgery, Sobell Department of Motor Neuroscience and Movement Disorders, Institute of Neurology, University College London, Box 146, Second Floor, 33 Queen Square, London, WC1N 3BG, UK
* Victor Horsley Department of Neurosurgery, National Hospital for Neurology and Neurosurgery, University College London Hospitals NHS Foundation Trust, Box 146, Second Floor, 33 Queen Square, London, WC1N 3BG, UK.
E-mail address: l.zrinzo@ion.ucl.ac.uk

Neuroimag Clin N Am 20 (2010) 125–140
doi:10.1016/j.nic.2009.08.002

lesions, but the incident highlighted the pallidum and thalamus as possible targets in PD.

The inconsistent results and high risk of vascular ablation pressed surgeons to develop alternative approaches. Probes were placed deep within the brain parenchyma via a burr hole under local anesthetic, initially guided solely by plain radiography and surgeon's intuition for anatomic localization.[27,28] Reversible lesions with local anesthetic or mild thermal manipulation allowed the effect of the intervention to be assessed before permanent chemical or thermal ablation. Despite functional improvements in individual patients, uncertainty about the anatomic location of the lesion interfered with replication of clinical results.[27] Clearly, a more reliable means of navigation within the brain was required.

The Stereotactic Technique

Precise neurosurgical targeting relies on the stereotactic technique, the principles of which were established by Clarke and Horsley in 1908.[29] "Stereotactic" literally means "three-dimensional touch," which conveys the philosophy behind this powerful navigational tool. It provides accurate localization of an intracranial target by ascertaining its triplanar coordinates with reference to fixed landmarks, and provides surgical access to targets deep within the brain in a minimally invasive fashion.

Historical inability to visualize the desired intracranial target led to the development of stereotactic atlases depicting the spatial relations of neural anatomy with respect to visible landmarks. At the beginning of the twentieth century, medical imaging technology was limited to Roentgen's development of radiographs in 1895.[30] The first stereotactic atlases therefore defined the spatial relations of cerebral structures with reference to bony landmarks. Considerable variability between bony cranial landmarks and enclosed neural structures severely limited the accuracy of such anatomic targeting.

Ventriculography and Its Legacy

The limited value of plain radiography in the localization of even large intracranial lesions drove Walter Dandy[31] to introduce air as a contrast medium outlining the ventricles as described in his seminal article of 1918.

Spiegel and colleagues[32] combined stereotactic principles with ventriculography to introduce the stereotactic technique to surgical practice in 1947. A frame applied to the skull provides visible external reference points to intracranial coordinates. The coordinates of intracerebral landmarks,

such as the anterior and posterior commissures (AC, PC), are acquired by imaging the patient's brain with the frame in situ. These neural landmarks enjoyed a much tighter spatial relation to the basal ganglia than did the bony landmarks of the cranium. Stereotactic atlases based on such neural landmarks therefore provide a more accurate method of anatomic localization, but do not eliminate the problem of anatomic variability completely. Nevertheless, the AC PC line still plays a central role in modern functional neurosurgical practice. In the 1950s and 1960s, the combination of the stereotactic technique, stereotactic atlases, and ventriculography allowed safe targeting of deep-seated structures, and the discipline of functional neurosurgery flourished.[33] Tens of thousands of patient with psychiatric and neurologic indications underwent functional neurosurgical operations in the years that followed. Cooper's service alone conducted almost 7000 functional interventions over 15 years.[28]

Refining of the Anatomic Target

Functional neurosurgical interventions are traditionally performed under local anesthesia. This technique allows surgeons to assess the clinical effects of the surgical intervention in "real time," in terms of the positive effect on symptoms and possible undesirable side effects. Diverse methods may be used to produce "reversible" lesions of the target area to assess the clinical effects, including thermal manipulation, injection of local anesthetic and high frequency electrical stimulation. Physiologic observations during surgery include measurement of electrical impedance and recording of neural activity (via micro- or macroelectrodes). These data allow functional neurosurgeons to corroborate the anatomic location of their surgical probe with physiologic and clinical findings.

Computerized Tomography and the Functional Hiatus

Functional surgery for motor disorders had become well established by the mid-1960s, but the number of procedures performed plummeted after the introduction of L-DOPA for the treatment of PD in 1967.[34] The introduction of pharmacologic means of treating psychiatric disorders, combined with the public backlash against flagrant abuse of surgical interventions by a few notorious but highly active individuals, led to the effective demise of psychiatric surgery.[35] Computerized tomography (CT) was introduced in the 1970s following the work of Hounsfield,[36] and allowed visualization of the AC and PC in a noninvasive fashion. However, the subspecialty field of functional neurosurgery had virtually come to a halt.[25,37]

RESURGENCE OF FUNCTIONAL NEUROSURGERY
Radiofrequency Thermal Lesions

During the last 2 decades of the twentieth century it became increasingly clear that medication was not the panacea it was initially believed to have been. Drug resistant symptoms, tolerance, and side effects led surgeons to re-explore the surgical approaches of earlier years. Laitinen's[38] seminal article revisiting Leksell's posteroventral radiofrequency pallidotomy was an important factor in this resurgence. Radiofrequency thermal lesions remain an excellent surgical technique offering a cheap and effective means of controlling the symptoms of various movement disorders at numerous brain targets.[38–42] The increased risk of adverse effects with bilateral basal ganglia lesions and their permanent nature have led to a decline in the use of this technique in favor of more modern alternatives.

New Technologies: Deep Brain Stimulation and Magnetic Resonance Imaging

Exploration of neural activity in the cortex and basal ganglia in health and disease suggested possible new targets for intervention, such as the subthalamic nucleus (STN) in PD, popularized by Benabid's group.[43] Fears of causing intolerable side effects provided the drive to commercially manufacture implantable hardware necessary for chronic high frequency stimulation of the brain.[40,44] Deep brain stimulation (DBS) has a similar functional effect to lesions but allows greater reversibility, flexibility, and adaptability than a permanent lesion. The most commonly used device for chronic DBS uses an implanted subclavian impulse generator (IPG) delivering variable monopolar or bipolar stimulation through any combination of 4 contacts at the end of a quadripolar electrode (**Fig. 1**).

Advances in imaging have had an immense impact on every branch of neurosurgery, and functional neurosurgery is no exception. With the resurgence of functional procedures, a few surgeons returned to the surgical approach of earlier years, relying on ventriculography and stereotactic atlases for their initial targeting. However, many surgeons turned toward the technological advances in axial imaging for initial anatomic targeting. Leksell,[45] with characteristic insight, recognized the fundamental importance of magnetic resonance imaging (MRI) in the practice of functional neurosurgery: "In clinical

practice, brain imaging can now be divided in two parts: the diagnostic neuroradiology and the preoperative stereotactic localization procedure. The latter is part of the therapeutic procedure. It is the surgeon's responsibility and should be closely integrated with the operation." The accuracy, speed and noninvasive nature of MRI compared with ventriculography is a major factor in its increasing use as the primary tool for anatomic targeting by functional neurosurgeons.[46,47] Nevertheless, several obstacles needed to be addressed before these advantages could be applied to clinical practice.

Structural Imaging

The tissue contrast visible within the brain parenchyma on early MR images was superior to that of CT but poor by modern standards. This limitation was rapidly addressed with advancing MR technology, higher field strengths, newer head coils, improved signal-to-noise ratios, and the introduction of a multitude of MR sequences that could be tailored to the area of interest.

The imaging protocols used in functional neurosurgery must establish a compromise between various factors. Target structures are often small, placing demands on image resolution. Visualization requires high tissue contrast between the target structure and the surrounding tissues. There is a limit to how long patients undergoing awake surgery can keep still in the MRI scanner, which places practical limits on image acquisition time. Acquired images should be contiguous thin slices. A voxel size of $1 \times 1 \times 2$ mm is often seen as an acceptable compromise between image resolution, signal-to-noise ratio, and practical image acquisition time on 1.5 T scanners. The publication of various imaging protocols that meet these criteria for specific anatomic targets allows for direct visualization on stereotactic MRI before surgical targeting (see later discussion).

Unlike diagnostic radiology, imaging for stereotactic surgery requires more than just visualization of structures. Inevitable inhomogeneities of the magnetic field can lead to geometric distortion of the acquired images.[48–50] This represents a significant obstacle to accurate spatial representation and can render such MR images useless for the purpose of accurate anatomic targeting (**Fig. 2**).

An increasingly popular approach is to address the issue of MR distortion directly.[49,51,52] Several methods for correction of field inhomogeneities have been described.[50,53–58] Manufacturers of MR scanners have incorporated software solutions that correct for distortion, resulting in

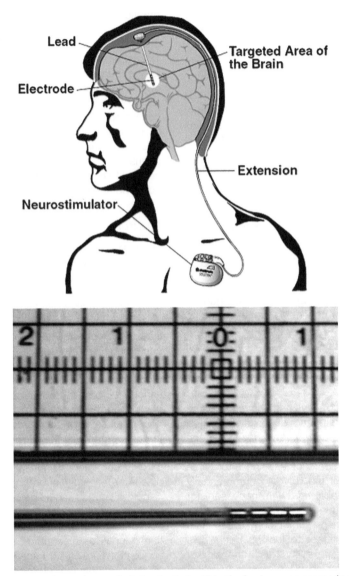

Fig.1. Implanted DBS system. Electrodes precisely implanted within the brain are connected to an implanted pulse generator via subcutaneous cables (*above*). Quadripolar electrode tip showing 4 contacts allowing monopolar or bipolar stimulation between contact and pulse generator case or between contact pairs respectively (*below*).

a greatly improved geometric accuracy of MR images. With adequate care and quality control, geometric errors can be reduced to the order of the pixel size and the submillimetre range.[59–65]

The use of stereotactic MRI in functional neurosurgery has practical implications for the design, structure, and application of the stereotactic frame. Evidently, the frame must be MR-compatible so that it exerts minimal distortion of the MR field.[66] Nevertheless, minimal geometric distortion can still be an issue close to the base of the frame. The surgeon should bear this in mind when applying the frame to the head such that the frame is as far away from the target region as possible.

Coronal images may suffer from greater distortion than axial images because the lower fiducials that lie close to the frame are required for stereotactic calculation on coronal images. It is therefore recommended that axial images are used in preference to coronal images when working with stereotactic MR images.

Geometric accuracy at the center of the MRI field tends to be excellent; however, distortion is exacerbated at the field periphery.[49,58,65,67] Therefore, frames with smaller fiducial indicator boxes (such as the Laitinen or Leksell systems) enjoy less geometric distortion than their larger counterparts. When preparing the patient for imaging, the

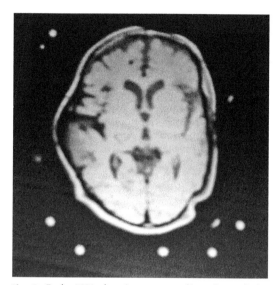

Fig. 2. Early MRI showing severe distortion of the brain and surrounding stereotactic fiducials. Numerous factors may contribute to image distortion. Attention to detail can avoid or correct for MR image distortion, allowing submillimetre accuracy in clinical practice (see text). (*Courtesy of* Marwan Hariz, Unit of Functional Neurosurgery, Queen Square, UCL, London, UK.)

surgeon should ensure that the radiographer advances the region of interest to the center of the magnetic field, as this tends to improve the geometric accuracy of the acquired images.[68] With adequate quality control it is becoming clear that MRI distortion need not be a clinically significant issue when used for anatomic targeting in functional neurosurgery.[66,69–73]

Another approach attempts to circumvent such problems by fusing or morphing nonstereotactic MR data onto stereotactic CT images, thus benefiting from contrast-rich MR data at the center of the field and the geometrically accurate fiducial localization of CT at the field periphery.[65,74–78] Numerous commercially available software packages now allow for this facility. However, this method remains prone to errors of image fusion that may ultimately dwarf the spatial errors introduced by MRI distortion.

Newer MR technologies result in fresh challenges: the faster and stronger gradient systems, shorter-bore magnets, and higher field strengths popular in modern magnets further compromise field homogeneity; however, awareness of the problem has led to innovative solutions.[51,79,80] Functional neurosurgery is renowned for its multidisciplinary nature, with excellent results being fostered in centers that enjoy close collaboration between neurologist and neurosurgeon. There is

no doubt that in the modern era, the MR physicist and neuroradiologist are key players in the multidisciplinary approach to functional neurosurgery. Imaging of the most popular and promising brain targets used in the surgical treatment of movement disorders is reviewed below.

Indirect Localization

Recognizing the AC and PC is an important step in indirect targeting. Once the AC, PC, and midcommissural points are defined in space, standard coordinates derived from stereotactic atlases can provide the surgeon with an estimated location of the target structure. Wherever possible, direct MRI visualization can then be used to refine the anatomic target.

The AC is a compact bundle of white matter connecting the olfactory and temporal regions of the 2 hemispheres.[81] Lying in the anterior wall of the third ventricle, 4 to 6 mm inferior to the foramen of Munro, it is often present on more than 1 axial image when contiguous 2-mm slices are acquired. Historically, it was the most posterior border of the AC that could be seen on ventriculography, and it is this point that should be defined on MR imaging (**Fig. 3**). The PC lies at the posterior aspect of the third ventricle and connects nuclei involved in eye movements and the pupillary light reflex.[81] On axial images, the third ventricle will be noted to have a box shape posteriorly. As one reaches the aqueduct, this box shape of the third ventricle disappears to give way to a funnel shape. The PC lies immediately rostral to the aqueduct and, on contiguous images, is therefore present on the most inferior axial slice before this narrowing occurs (see **Fig. 3**). The AC and PC are best defined on T1-weighted MR images. The PC may occasionally be difficult to discern, especially on CT images of younger patients with narrow third ventricles.

Standard coordinates give an estimate of the location of surgically relevant targets in relation to the midcommissural point. Anatomic variability results in diverse coordinates being quoted for the same structures. The present author uses the following coordinates from the midcommissural point for initial indirect localization and refines these further by direct visualization of the target structure wherever possible: STN: 12 mm lateral, 2 mm posterior, 5 mm inferior; posteroventral pallidum: 21 mm lateral, 2 mm anterior, 5mm inferior; motor thalamus: 13 to 15 mm lateral, 6 mm posterior, at the level of the AC PC plane.

The use of commercially available planning software allows planning of target and trajectory. Planned trajectories that avoid the cerebral sulci and ventricles would avoid the intrasulcal and

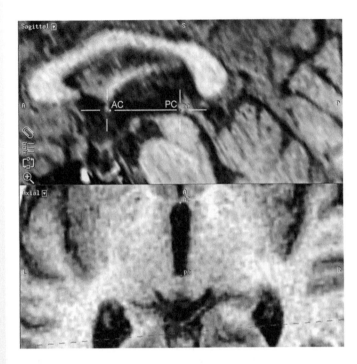

Fig. 3. The stereotactic location of anatomic structures can be estimated from their relation to internal landmarks as defined by stereotactic atlases. The AC and PC are the most commonly used internal landmarks and can be defined on ventriculography, CT, and MRI. T1-weighted MRI: midline sagittal reconstruction (*top*) and axial image in the commissural plane. Note the squared-off posterior aspect of the third ventricle at the level of the PC. A funnel appearance of the posterior aspect of the third ventricle suggests visualization of the aqueduct that lies below the level of the PC.

intraventricular vessels, theoretically minimizing the risk of hemorrhage.

Direct Localization

STN

The STN is a popular and effective target in the symptomatic management of PD. Models of information flow through the basal ganglia suggest that this nucleus is overactive in PD with abnormal synchronization of neuronal activity in the beta range (13–30 Hz).[82] Lesioning or chronic high-frequency stimulation of this nucleus is believed to disrupt abnormal neuronal activity and restore some balance to the corticobasal ganglia circuitry involved in control of movement.[83] Tens of thousands of patients have undergone STN DBS with, on the whole, beneficial effects on bradykinesia, rigidity, tremor, and motor fluctuations.

Located in the rostral mesencephalon, the STN is a small biconvex structure (3 × 5 × 12 mm) lying posteromedial to the crus cerebri; its longitudinal axis is obliquely oriented such that the superior pole lies lateral and posterior to the inferior one.[81,84–86] Functional segregation of the nucleus into motor, cognitive, and limbic portions mirrors that of other basal ganglia structures. Extrapolation from animal studies and MRI localization of the most effective active DBS contacts suggest that the motor component of the STN is located in its most superior portion.[86–88]

The STN can be visualized on MRI, allowing direct targeting of this structure (**Fig. 4**).[47,84,89,90] On T2-weighted images, the STN presents a characteristic hypointense signal that has been attributed to the presence of iron.[91–93] Bejjani and colleagues[84] proposed the red nuclei as an internal landmark to the STN (see **Fig. 4**). Concerns have been raised about discrepancies between the expected size of the STN on MRI and that seen on histologic atlases.[94] This may represent a relative paucity of iron deposits within the posterior portion of the nucleus, thus rendering part of the nucleus less visible on MRI.[91] Nonetheless, stereotactic localization is better served by direct visualization of part of the target structure than by estimating its location based on stereotactic atlases.

Globus pallidus internus

Forming the most medial part of the lentiform nucleus, the globus pallidus internus (GPi) lies medial to the lamina interna and lateral to the internal capsule.[81] Numerous investigators targeted the ansa lenticularis and pallidum in the early decades of the twentieth century, with Leksell noting superior results in the posteroventral region.[24,95,96] Motor function was later mapped to the posteroventral portion of the GPi in animal studies, confirming Leksell's clinical observations, and this is now the accepted surgical target in the treatment of various dystonias and dyskinesia.[3,38,97–99]

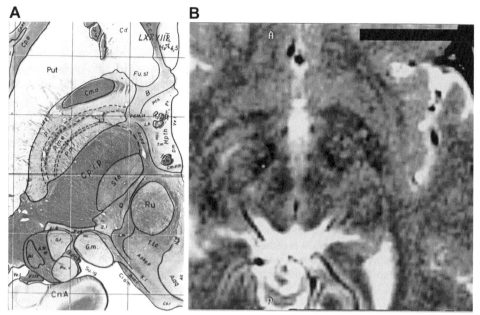

Fig. 4. (A) Histologic section taken 4.5 mm below the midcommissural point. Note the round red nucleus (Ru) and its relation to the biconvex STN. (B) Axial image taken from T2-weighted stereotactic MRI (1.5 T). The red nuclei can be seen as round hypointense signals anterolateral to the aqueduct. The STN can be visualized as the ovoid hypointensity lying anterolateral to the red nucleus, with its long axis lying oblique to the midline. (From Schaltenbrand G, Wahren W. Atlas for stereotaxy of the human brainsecond edition, revised and enlarged. Chicago: Year Book Medical Publishers; 1977. Plate 29; with permission.)

MRI protocols that allow clear visualization of the pallidal architecture have been published.[100–102] The author uses a modified proton-density sequence for targeting the posteroventral pallidum (Fig. 5). The putamen, internal and external pallidum, and the pallidocapsular border can easily be seen at the level of the AC. This sequence guides the surgical trajectory to the posteroventral pallidum as it lies immediately superior and lateral to the optic tract.

Motor thalamus and zona incerta
The motor thalamus (Vim, Vop and Voa/VLp: Hassler/Hirai and Jones classifications respectively) is

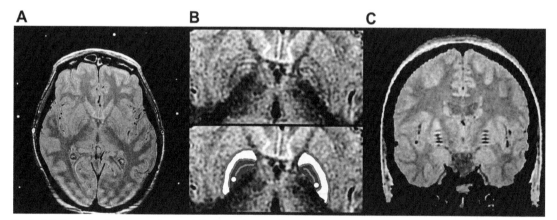

Fig. 5. (A) Stereotactic proton-density MRI in patient undergoing pallidal DBS for dystonia. (B) (top and bottom) Lentiform nuclei at the level of the AC. The lateral and medial medullary laminae separate putamen, external pallidum (white crescent), and internal pallidum (gray). The small accessory lamina that bisects the internal pallidum can also be visualized. The posterior part of the internal pallidum that is targeted in the treatment of dystonias and dyskinesias is marked with a small white circle. (C) The DBS electrode is directed inferiorly to reach the most posteroventral part of the GPi. The artifacts left by the quadripolar electrodes can be seen lying lateral and medial to the optic tract on the coronal image on the right.

an excellent surgical target for addressing tremor.[103] Visualization of individual thalamic nuclei is unreliable at 1.5 T although attempts have been made to visualize these at higher field strengths.[104–107] Indirect targeting currently retains an important role in the use of this target, although the lateral and anteroposterior coordinates can be guided by visualization of the thalamocapsular border on CT or MRI.

The zona incerta (ZI) is continuous with the inferior aspect of the thalamic reticular nucleus, and has been proposed as an alternative target to motor thalamus and STN for tremor and parkinsonism respectively.[108–110] Lying on the superomedial aspect of the STN, and medial to its most superior and lateral tail, direct ZI localization is possible on T2-weighted scans (**Fig. 6**). It is usually possible to plan a trajectory that will allow a quadripolar DBS electrode to straddle ZI and motor thalamic targets.

Pedunculopontine nucleus

The pedunculopontine nucleus (PPN) forms part of the rostral locomotor region of the brainstem and is believed to play a central role in the initiation and maintenance of gait.[111] An elongated neuronal collection in the lateral pontine and mesencephalic tegmental reticular zones, the nucleus straddles the pontomesencephalic junction, its long axis roughly parallel to that of the fourth ventricle floor.[112] The rostral pole lies at midinferior collicular level, the nucleus extending circa 5 mm caudally to reach the rostral pons.[113,114] A triad of projection pathways circumscribes the region of the PPN: the superior cerebellar peduncle and its decussation, the central tegmental tract, and the lemniscal system (**Fig. 7**). Translational research has led to promising reports of DBS in the rostral brainstem in humans.[115–117] However, this region of the brain is unfamiliar territory to most functional neurosurgeons, and has been the subject of inaccurate descriptions and representations.[118–121] Images acquired using a specifically modified proton-density MRI protocol provide excellent definition between gray and white matter within the region of interest at 1.5 T.[100] This method, together with an understanding of the regional anatomy, allows accurate PPN localization on stereotactic MRI in clinical practice (see **Fig. 7**).[122]

Tractography

Diffusion tensor imaging and tractography have been used as research tools to examine the connectivity of the intended targets for surgical intervention and the theoretical spread of current from active DBS contacts.[123–126] More recently, it has been suggested that the information provided by tractography may be used in defining the surgical target.[127–129] This imaging technique tends to use a large voxel size. In addition, a somewhat arbitrary level of significance is assigned to the process of defining a fiber tract by anisotropy. These issues require further attention to allow the practical use of this technique by functional neurosurgeons.

Documentation of Electrode Localization

Accuracy and precision of electrode placement is of great importance in functional neurosurgery, and surgeons therefore place great emphasis on preoperative imaging and targeting.[130,131] Equal efforts should be made to verify that the target area has been reached. The gold standard in this verification process is postoperative MR stereotactic imaging localizing the implanted electrodes within the preoperatively defined stereotactic space.[132,133] This also allows documentation of complications such as hemorrhage. Failing this, postoperative stereotactic radiography or CT will also allow an assessment of electrode contact location in stereotactic space.[134] Fusion to a preoperative MRI will allow estimation of contact location in relation to anatomic

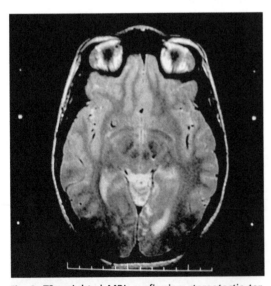

Fig. 6. T2-weighted MRI confirming stereotactic targeting of the ZI lying posteromedial to the lateral tail of the STN in a patient with unilateral tremor. Note the hyperintense stereotactic fiducials surrounding the head. The signal void artifact of the DBS electrode; the characteristic hyperintense signal posterior to the electrode artifact that should not be confused with hemorrhage.

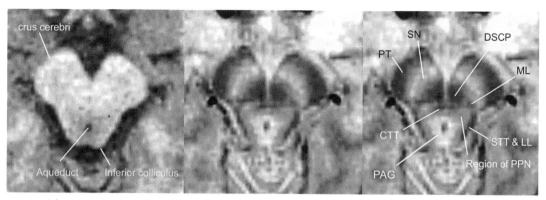

Fig. 7. Axial MRI images through the inferior colliculi. The T1 image on the left shows excellent contrast between brain and CSF, but little internal tissue contrast. The proton-density MRI sequence from the same patient provides excellent tissue contrast: gray matter appears hyperintense (*bright*); white matter appears hypointense (*dark*). Identifiable anatomic structures are labeled on the right. Note how the region of the PPN is of intermediate density between that of gray matter (eg, PAG) and white matter (eg, DSCP) perhaps in view of its reticular nature. CTT, central tegmental tract; DSCP, decussation of the superior cerebellar peduncles; LL, lateral lemniscus; ML, medial lemniscus; PAG, periaqueductal gray; PPN, pedunculopontine nucleus; PT, pyramidal tract; SN, substantia nigra; STT, spinothalamic tract. (*From* Zrinzo L, Zrinzo LV, Tisch S, et al. Stereotactic localization of the human pedunculopontine nucleus: atlas-based coordinates and validation of a magnetic resonance imaging protocol for direct localization. Brain 2008;131:1588; with permission.)

structures. The imaging characteristics of commercially available electrodes has been determined on CT and MR.[134,135] The MRI artifact is larger than the electrode itself, and a hyperintensity may be seen around the electrode tip that should not be confused with hemorrhage (see **Fig. 6**).

Several investigators have addressed the issue of documenting electrode location.[71,87,88,131,134,136–141] Attention to the details of anatomic targeting as described above can achieve impressive degrees of accuracy. The mean (SD) targeting error at the author's institution is 1.0 (0.5) mm (unpublished data). Increased anatomic targeting accuracy seems to significantly reduce the need for multiple brain passes to achieve the desired target, as defined by clinical and physiologic observations.[142] Indeed, some groups believe that anatomic targeting accuracy is so reliable that they advocate placement of DBS electrodes under general anesthesia, with immediate confirmation of lead location on stereotactic MRI.[131] This approach does away with intraoperative clinical and physiologic observations, traditionally a central tenet of functional neurosurgery. However, it allows for surgical intervention on patients who would otherwise not be suitable for local anesthesia (eg, children, patients whose symptoms render surgery under local anesthesia impractical). The author has used this approach to good effect with various anatomic targets including the GPi and STN.

Radiosurgery

Image-guided radiosurgery may also be used to create stereotactic lesions in a noninvasive fashion.[96] However, there are many disadvantages of using this approach. Radiosurgery acts in a delayed fashion by causing avascular necrosis of the targeted region. The effects are therefore delayed and the ultimate size of the lesion difficult to control.[143] In addition, the inability to modulate the therapy based on clinical and physiologic observations before inflicting a permanent lesion does not rest easy with the philosophy of this discipline. Radiosurgical Vim thalamotomy may still be an option in a small subgroup of patients with tremor whose age, comorbidity, or coagulation status prohibit open surgery.[144]

Functional Imaging

Functional imaging of brain activity using positron emission tomography (PET) and functional MRI (fMRI) has been of practical use in functional neurosurgery. Functional imaging has revealed regions of overactivity in conditions such as cluster headache (the posterior hypothalamus)[145,146] and depression (the subgenual cingulate gyrus).[16,147] This has provided theoretical impetus to the implantation of DBS electrodes within these regions, and has provided relief in some patients with previously intractable symptoms.[16,148,149] Functional imaging has also been used as a research tool to shed light on the physiologic mechanisms that underlie the clinical improvements seen with DBS.[150–153]

Safety Issues

MR imaging of the brain after electrode implantation is of paramount importance. The potential risks of performing MRI examinations with implanted DBS hardware include induction of electrical currents, magnetic field interactions, interference with DBS hardware, and local heating. Isolated reports of neurologic deterioration after MRI have been published.[154,155]

Following these reports, the manufacturer updated the safety guidelines (November 2005),[156] requiring: (1) that the device be turned off, with amplitude at zero in bipolar mode; (2) the use of a T/R head coil that does not extend over the chest (IPG) area; (3) the limiting of the displayed average specific absorption rate (SAR) on the MR console to less than or equal to 0.1 W/kg (down from the previous figure of ≤0.4 W/kg in previous guidelines).

Restricting SAR in MRI systems limits heat deposition in tissues. MRI scanners use "predictive models" that vary between manufacturers and even software versions on the same scanner. This variation makes SAR a poor predictor for potential heating effects near DBS leads, but at present it is the only measure available.[157] Phantom studies have shown that SAR is not the only determinant of tissue heating and that head transmit/receive coils result in much less heating than their body counterparts at the same displayed average SAR.[158] They also demonstrated clinically acceptable levels of heating (<0.5°C) with SAR values of 0.5 W/kg.[159] More recent phantom studies suggest that at 1.5 T and 3 T, given adequate precautions, fMRI studies can be performed at SAR values of ≤0.4 W/kg with no measurable temperature change even if the device is switched on (<0.1°C).[160]

Larson and colleagues[157] provide an excellent review of the safety of MRI events in patients with implanted DBS hardware. They present their extensive MRI experience at 1.5 T with SAR of up to 3 W/kg for a total of 1071 MRI events with no adverse events, and conclude that "the 0.1 W/kg recommended safety margin for SAR, which is impractical for high-quality imaging, may be unnecessarily low for prevention of MRI-related adverse events."[157] Experience in our institution mirrors these findings, with MRI being conducted in more than 200 patients with implanted DBS hardware without adverse events using average SAR values of less than or equal to 0.4 W/kg over the last 6 years. The authors use the added precaution of video camera surveillance, ensuring that the patient does not move the head during image acquisition.

One group has circumvented these safety issues by developing custom-made plastic guide tubes with a radio-opaque stylette allowing perioperative radiological confirmation of location. Withdrawal of the stylette allows the guide tube to act as a port for the implantation of an electrode for DBS.[131]

New Challenges

The rapid pace of development of MR technologies and their swift dissemination into clinical practice opens new horizons in functional neurosurgery. High field imaging, new head coils, and novel imaging sequences promise enhanced tissue contrast, finer image resolution, and faster scanning times (Fig. 8). Anatomic structures are being visualized in vivo with hitherto unimaginable

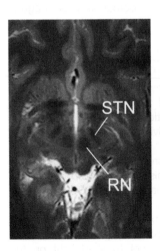

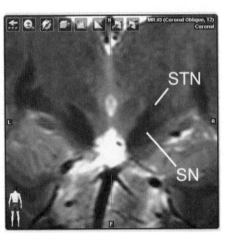

Fig. 8. MR images at 7 T. Axial T2 image reveals the red nuclei and subthalamic nuclei in exquisite detail. Note the slight asymmetry between the 2 sides. Coronal images clearly show the subthalamic nuclei lying superior to the substantia nigra. STN, subthalamic nucleus; SN, substantia nigra. (Courtesy of Hans Hoogduin, Fredy Visser, Peter Luijten, Division of RRN and Brain Division, UMC Utrecht, The Netherlands and Arjen van Hulzen, Michiel Staal, Department of Neurosurgery, UMC Groningen, The Netherlands.)

detail; this places even greater emphasis on the need to determine the histologic correlates of MR images. Techniques such as fMRI, Doppler tissue imaging (DTI), and magnetoencephalography (MEG) may help shed light on the mechanisms by which DBS exerts its beneficial effects, or may even suggest new therapeutic targets. Yet these advances bring with them new challenges that must be overcome before these advantages can be harnessed in a clinically relevant fashion. Higher field strengths and shorter scanner bores are liable to even greater safety and image distortion issues. There is no doubt that imaging will continue to play an ever increasing role in functional neurosurgery, and multidisciplinary groups are best placed to maximize its potential.

SUMMARY

Modern neurosurgical practice is inextricably linked to technological advances in medical imaging. From its conception, advances in the surgical treatment of movement disorders have been intertwined with developments in medical imaging.

Meticulous attention to detail is required during image acquisition, direct anatomic localization, and planning of the initial surgical trajectory. This approach may allow the surgeon to reach the desired anatomic and functional target with the initial trajectory in most cases, minimizing the need for multiple passes through the brain and the associated risk of hemorrhage and functional deficit. This philosophy is of paramount importance in a procedure that is primarily aimed at improving quality of life. Finally, documentation of electrode contact location by means of stereotactic imaging is essential to audit surgical targeting accuracy and to further our knowledge of structure-to-function relationships within the human brain.

REFERENCES

1. Limousin P, Pollak P, Benazzouz A, et al. Effect of parkinsonian signs and symptoms of bilateral subthalamic nucleus stimulation. Lancet 1995;345: 91–5.
2. Schüpbach WM, Maltête D, Houeto JL, et al. Neurosurgery at an earlier stage of Parkinson disease: a randomized, controlled trial. Neurology 2007;68:267–71.
3. Coubes P, Roubertie A, Vayssiere N, et al. Treatment of DYT1-generalised dystonia by stimulation of the internal globus pallidus. Lancet 2000;355: 2220–1.
4. Hung SW, Hamani C, Lozano AM, et al. Long-term outcome of bilateral pallidal deep brain stimulation for primary cervical dystonia. Neurology 2007;68:457–9.
5. Hariz GM, Lindberg M, Bergenheim AT. Impact of thalamic deep brain stimulation on disability and health-related quality of life in patients with essential tremor. J Neurol Neurosurg Psychiatry 2002; 72:47–52.
6. Rehncrona S, Johnels B, Widner H, et al. Long-term efficacy of thalamic deep brain stimulation for tremor: double-blind assessments. Mov Disord 2003;18:163–70.
7. Cruccu G, Aziz TZ, Garcia-Larrea L, et al. EFNS guidelines on neurostimulation therapy for neuropathic pain. Eur J Neurol 2007;14:952–70.
8. Levy RM. Deep brain stimulation for the treatment of intractable pain. Neurosurg Clin N Am 2003;14: 389–99.
9. Leone M, Franzini A, Bussone G. Stereotactic stimulation of posterior hypothalamic gray matter in a patient with intractable cluster headache. N Engl J Med 2001;345:1428–9.
10. Servello D, Porta M, Sassi M, et al. Deep brain stimulation in 18 patients with severe Gilles de la Tourette syndrome refractory to treatment: the surgery and stimulation. J Neurol Neurosurg Psychiatry 2008;79:136–42.
11. Temel Y, Visser-Vandewalle V. Surgery in Tourette syndrome. Mov Disord 2004;19:3–14.
12. Welter ML, Mallet L, Houeto JL, et al. Internal pallidal and thalamic stimulation in patients with Tourette syndrome. Arch Neurol 2008;65:952–7.
13. Cosgrove GR, Rauch SL. Stereotactic cingulotomy. Neurosurg Clin N Am 2003;14:225–35.
14. Eljamel MS. Ablative neurosurgery for mental disorders: is there still a role in the 21st century? A personal perspective. Neurosurg Focus 2008;25: E4.
15. Greenberg BD, Malone DA, Friehs GM, et al. Three-year outcomes in deep brain stimulation for highly resistant obsessive-compulsive disorder. Neuropsychopharmacology 2006;31:2384–93.
16. Lozano AM, Mayberg HS, Giacobbe P, et al. Subcallosal cingulate gyrus deep brain stimulation for treatment-resistant depression. Biol Psychiatry 2008;64:461–7.
17. Andrade DM, Zumsteg D, Hamani C, et al. Long-term follow-up of patients with thalamic deep brain stimulation for epilepsy. Neurology 2006; 66:1571–3.
18. Velasco AL, Velasco F, Velasco M, et al. Electrical stimulation of the hippocampal epileptic foci for seizure control: a double-blind, long-term follow-up study. Epilepsia 2007;48:1895–903.
19. Velasco F, Velasco AL, Velasco M, et al. Deep brain stimulation for treatment of the epilepsies: the

centromedian thalamic target. Acta Neurochir Suppl 2007;97:337–42.

20. Horsley V. The Linacre Lecture on the function of the so-called motor area of the brain. Br Med J 1909;2:125–32.

21. Horsley V. Remarks on the surgery of the central nervous system. Br Med J 1890;2:1286–92.

22. Putnam TJ. Treatment of athetosis and dystonia by section of extrapyramidal motor tracts. Arch Neurol Psychiatry 1933;29:504–21.

23. Meyers R. Surgical experiments in the therapy of certain 'extrapyramidal' diseases: a current evaluation. Acta Psychiatr Neurol Suppl 1951;67:1–42.

24. Meyers R. Surgical procedure for postencephalitic tremor, with notes on the physiology of premotor fibers. Arch Neurol Psychiatry 1940;44:455–9.

25. Gildenberg PL. The history of surgery for movement disorders. Neurosurg Clin N Am 1998;9:283–94.

26. Cooper IS. Ligation of the anterior choroidal artery for involuntary movements; parkinsonism. Psychiatr Q 1953;27:317–9.

27. Cooper IS. The vital probe: my life as an experimental brain surgeon. 1st edition. New York: Norton; 1981.

28. Cooper IS. Involuntary movement disorders. New York: Hoeber Medical Division; 1969.

29. Horsley V, Clarke RH. The structure and functions of the cerebellum examined by a new method. Brain 1908;31:45–124.

30. Röntgen WK. On a new kind of rays. Nature 1896; 53:274–6.

31. Dandy WE. Ventriculography following the injection of air into the cerebral ventricles. Ann Surg 1918; 68:5–11.

32. Spiegel EA, Wycis HT, Marks M, et al. Stereotaxic apparatus for operations on the human brain. Science 1947;106:349–50.

33. Hassler R, Riechert T. A special method of stereotactic brain operation. Proc R Soc Med 1955;48: 469–70.

34. Cotzias GC, Van Woert MH, Schiffer LM. Aromatic amino acids and modification of parkinsonism. N Engl J Med 1967;276:374–9.

35. Hariz MI. Psychosurgery, deep brain stimulation, and the re-writing of history. Neurosurgery 2008; 63:E820 author reply E820.

36. Hounsfield GN. Computerized transverse axial scanning (tomography). 1. Description of system. Br J Radiol 1973;46:1016–22.

37. Gildenberg PL. Whatever happened to stereotactic surgery? Neurosurgery 1987;20:983–7.

38. Laitinen LV, Bergenheim AT, Hariz MI. Leksell's posteroventral pallidotomy in the treatment of Parkinson's disease. J Neurosurg 1992;76:53–61.

39. Alvarez L, Macias R, Lopez G, et al. Bilateral subthalamotomy in Parkinson's disease: initial and long-term response. Brain 2005;128:570–83.

40. Benabid AL, Pollak P, Louveau A, et al. Combined (thalamotomy and stimulation) stereotactic surgery of the VIM thalamic nucleus for bilateral Parkinson disease. Appl Neurophysiol 1987;50:344–6.

41. Blomstedt P, Hariz GM, Hariz MI. Pallidotomy versus pallidal stimulation. Parkinsonism Relat Disord 2006;12:296–301.

42. Taira T, Hori T. Stereotactic ventrooralis thalamotomy for task-specific focal hand dystonia (writer's cramp). Stereotact Funct Neurosurg 2003;80:88–91.

43. Limousin P, Krack P, Pollak P, et al. Electrical stimulation of the subthalamic nucleus in advanced Parkinson's disease. N Engl J Med 1998;339:1105–11.

44. Bechtereva NP, Bondartchuk AN, Smirnov VM, et al. Method of electrostimulation of the deep brain structures in treatment of some chronic diseases. Confin Neurol 1975;37:136–40.

45. Leksell L, Leksell D, Schwebel J. Stereotaxis and nuclear magnetic resonance. J Neurol Neurosurg Psychiatry 1985;48:14–8.

46. Hariz MI, Bergenheim AT. A comparative study on ventriculographic and computerized tomography-guided determinations of brain targets in functional stereotaxis. J Neurosurg 1990;73:565–71.

47. Schuurman PR, de Bie RM, Majoie CB, et al. A prospective comparison between three-dimensional magnetic resonance imaging and ventriculography for target-coordinate determination in frame-based functional stereotactic neurosurgery. J Neurosurg 1999;91:911–4.

48. O'Donnell M, Edelstein WA. NMR imaging in the presence of magnetic field inhomogeneities and gradient field nonlinearities. Med Phys 1985;12:20–6.

49. Sumanaweera TS, Adler JR Jr, Napel S, et al. Characterization of spatial distortion in magnetic resonance imaging and its implications for stereotactic surgery. Neurosurgery 1994;35:696–703.

50. Sumanaweera TS, Glover GH, Binford TO, et al. MR susceptibility misregistration correction. IEEE Trans Med Imaging 1993;12:251–9.

51. Doran SJ, Charles-Edwards L, Reinsberg SA, et al. A complete distortion correction for MR images: I. Gradient warp correction. Phys Med Biol 2005;50: 1343–61.

52. Reinsberg SA, Doran SJ, Charles-Edwards EM, et al. A complete distortion correction for MR images: II. Rectification of static-field inhomogeneities by similarity-based profile mapping. Phys Med Biol 2005;50:2651–61.

53. Bakker CJ, Moerland MA, Bhagwandien R, et al. Analysis of machine-dependent and object-induced geometric distortion in 2DFT MR imaging. Magn Reson Imaging 1992;10:597–608.

54. Chang H, Fitzpatrick JM. A technique for accurate magnetic resonance imaging in the presence of

field inhomogeneities. IEEE Trans Med Imaging 1992;11:319–29.

55. Jones AP. Diagnostic imaging as a measuring device for stereotactic neurosurgery. Physiol Meas 1993;14:91–112.

56. Moerland MA, Beersma R, Bhagwandien R, et al. Analysis and correction of geometric distortions in 1.5 T magnetic resonance images for use in radiotherapy treatment planning. Phys Med Biol 1995; 40:1651–4.

57. Schad LR, Ehricke HH, Wowra B, et al. Correction of spatial distortion in magnetic resonance angiography for radiosurgical treatment planning of cerebral arteriovenous malformations. Magn Reson Imaging 1992;10:609–21.

58. Sumanaweera TS, Adler JR, Glover GH, et al. Method for correcting magnetic resonance image distortion for frame-based stereotactic surgery, with preliminary results. J Image Guid Surg 1995; 1:151–7.

59. Bednarz G, Downes MB, Corn BW, et al. Evaluation of the spatial accuracy of magnetic resonance imaging-based stereotactic target localization for gamma knife radiosurgery of functional disorders. Neurosurgery 1999;45:1156–61.

60. Bourgeois G, Magnin M, Morel A, et al. Accuracy of MRI-guided stereotactic thalamic functional neurosurgery. Neuroradiology 1999;41:636–45.

61. Hirabayashi H, Hariz MI, Fagerlund M. Comparison between stereotactic CT and MRI coordinates of pallidal and thalamic targets using the Laitinen noninvasive stereoadapter. Stereotact Funct Neurosurg 1998;71:117–30.

62. Walton L, Hampshire A, Forster DM, et al. Stereotactic localization with magnetic resonance imaging: a phantom study to compare the accuracy obtained using two-dimensional and three-dimensional data acquisitions. Neurosurgery 1997;41:131–7.

63. Wu TH, Lee JS, Wu HM, et al. Evaluating geometric accuracy of multi-platform stereotactic neuroimaging in radiosurgery. Stereotact Funct Neurosurg 2002;78:39–48.

64. Yu C, Apuzzo ML, Zee CS, et al. A phantom study of the geometric accuracy of computed tomographic and magnetic resonance imaging stereotactic localization with the Leksell stereotactic system. Neurosurgery 2001;48:1092–8.

65. Yu C, Petrovich Z, Apuzzo ML, et al. An image fusion study of the geometric accuracy of magnetic resonance imaging with the Leksell stereotactic localization system. J Appl Clin Med Phys 2001;2: 42–50.

66. Burchiel KJ, Nguyen TT, Coombs BD, et al. MRI distortion and stereotactic neurosurgery using the Cosman-Roberts-Wells and Leksell frames. Stereotact Funct Neurosurg 1996;66:123–36.

67. Sumanaweera T, Glover G, Song S, et al. Quantifying MRI geometric distortion in tissue. Magn Reson Med 1994;31:40–7.

68. Guo WY, Chu WC, Wu MC, et al. An evaluation of the accuracy of magnetic-resonance-guided gamma knife surgery. Stereotact Funct Neurosurg 1996;66(Suppl 1):85–92.

69. Carter DA, Parsai EI, Ayyangar KM. Accuracy of magnetic resonance imaging stereotactic coordinates with the Cosman-Roberts-Wells frame. Stereotact Funct Neurosurg 1999;72:35–46.

70. Landi A, Marina R, DeGrandi C, et al. Accuracy of stereotactic localisation with magnetic resonance compared to CT scan: experimental findings. Acta Neurochir (Wien) 2001;143:593–607.

71. Martin AJ, Larson PS, Ostrem JL, et al. Placement of deep brain stimulator electrodes using real-time high-field interventional magnetic resonance imaging. Magn Reson Med 2005;54: 1107–14.

72. Menuel C, Garnero L, Bardinet E, et al. Characterization and correction of distortions in stereotactic magnetic resonance imaging for bilateral subthalamic stimulation in Parkinson disease. J Neurosurg 2005;103:256–66.

73. Simon SL, Douglas P, Baltuch GH, et al. Error analysis of MRI and Leksell stereotactic frame target localization in deep brain stimulation surgery. Stereotact Funct Neurosurg 2005;83:1–5.

74. Alexander E 3rd, Kooy HM, van Herk M, et al. Magnetic resonance image-directed stereotactic neurosurgery: use of image fusion with computerized tomography to enhance spatial accuracy. J Neurosurg 1995;83:271–6.

75. Aziz TZ, Nandi D, Parkin S, et al. Targeting the subthalamic nucleus. Stereotact Funct Neurosurg 2001;77:87–90.

76. Holtzheimer PE 3rd, Roberts DW, Darcey TM. Magnetic resonance imaging versus computed tomography for target localization in functional stereotactic neurosurgery. Neurosurgery 1999;45: 290–7.

77. Kondziolka D, Dempsey PK, Lunsford LD, et al. A comparison between magnetic resonance imaging and computed tomography for stereotactic coordinate determination. Neurosurgery 1992;30:402–6.

78. Wyper DJ, Turner JW, Patterson J, et al. Accuracy of stereotaxic localisation using MRI and CT. J Neurol Neurosurg Psychiatry 1986;49:1445–8.

79. Wang D, Doddrell DM. Method for a detailed measurement of image intensity nonuniformity in magnetic resonance imaging. Med Phys 2005;32: 952–60.

80. Wang D, Doddrell DM, Cowin G. A novel phantom and method for comprehensive 3-dimensional measurement and correction of geometric

distortion in magnetic resonance imaging. Magn Reson Imaging 2004;22:529–42.

81. Parent A, Carpenter MB. Human neuroanatomy. 9th edition. Baltimore (MD): Williams & Wilkins; 1995.

82. Brown P. Bad oscillations in Parkinson's disease. J Neural Transm Suppl 2006;27–30.

83. Kühn AA, Kempf F, Brücke C, et al. High-frequency stimulation of the subthalamic nucleus suppresses oscillatory beta activity in patients with Parkinson's disease in parallel with improvement in motor performance. J Neurosci 2008;28:6165–73.

84. Bejjani BP, Dormont D, Pidoux B, et al. Bilateral subthalamic stimulation for Parkinson's disease by using three-dimensional stereotactic magnetic resonance imaging and electrophysiological guidance. J Neurosurg 2000;92:615–25.

85. Yelnik J. Functional anatomy of the basal ganglia. Mov Disord 2002;17(Suppl 3):S15–21.

86. Yelnik J, Bardinet E, Dormont D, et al. A three-dimensional, histological and deformable atlas of the human basal ganglia. I. Atlas construction based on immunohistochemical and MRI data. Neuroimage 2007;34:618–38.

87. Chen CC, Pogosyan A, Zrinzo LU, et al. Intra-operative recordings of local field potentials can help localize the subthalamic nucleus in Parkinson's disease surgery. Exp Neurol 2006;198:214–21.

88. Saint-Cyr JA, Hoque T, Pereira LC, et al. Localization of clinically effective stimulating electrodes in the human subthalamic nucleus on magnetic resonance imaging. J Neurosurg 2002;97:1152–66.

89. Hariz MI, Krack P, Melvill R, et al. A quick and universal method for stereotactic visualization of the subthalamic nucleus before and after implantation of deep brain stimulation electrodes. Stereotact Funct Neurosurg 2003;80:96–101.

90. Voges J, Volkmann J, Allert N, et al. Bilateral high-frequency stimulation in the subthalamic nucleus for the treatment of Parkinson disease: correlation of therapeutic effect with anatomical electrode position. J Neurosurg 2002;96:269–79.

91. Dormont D, Ricciardi KG, Tande D, et al. Is the subthalamic nucleus hypointense on T2-weighted images? A correlation study using MR imaging and stereotactic atlas data. AJNR Am J Neuroradiol 2004;25:1516–23.

92. Drayer B, Burger P, Darwin R, et al. MRI of brain iron. AJR Am J Roentgenol 1986;147:103–10.

93. Drayer B, Burger P, Hurwitz B, et al. Reduced signal intensity on MR images of thalamus and putamen in multiple sclerosis: increased iron content? AJR Am J Roentgenol 1987;149:357–63.

94. Richter EO, Hoque T, Halliday W, et al. Determining the position and size of the subthalamic nucleus based on magnetic resonance imaging results in patients with advanced Parkinson disease. J Neurosurg 2004;100:541–6.

95. Narabayashi H, Okuma T, Shikiba S. Procaine oil blocking of the globus pallidus. AMA Arch Neurol Psychiatry 1956;75:36–48.

96. Svennilson E, Torvik A, Lowe R, et al. Treatment of parkinsonism by stereotatic thermolesions in the pallidal region. A clinical evaluation of 81 cases. Acta Psychiatr Scand 1960;35:358–77.

97. Parent A, De Bellefeuille L. Organization of efferent projections from the internal segment of globus pallidus in primate as revealed by fluorescence retrograde labeling method. Brain Res 1982;245:201–13.

98. Tisch S, Zrinzo L, Limousin P, et al. Effect of electrode contact location on clinical efficacy of pallidal deep brain stimulation in primary generalised dystonia. J Neurol Neurosurg Psychiatry 2007;78:1314–9.

99. Yelnik J, Damier P, Bejjani BP, et al. Functional mapping of the human globus pallidus: contrasting effect of stimulation in the internal and external pallidum in Parkinson's disease. Neuroscience 2000;101:77–87.

100. Hirabayashi H, Tengvar M, Hariz MI. Stereotactic imaging of the pallidal target. Mov Disord 2002;17(Suppl 3):S130–4.

101. Vayssiere N, Hemm S, Cif L, et al. Comparison of atlas- and magnetic resonance imaging-based stereotactic targeting of the globus pallidus internus in the performance of deep brain stimulation for treatment of dystonia. J Neurosurg 2002;96:673–9.

102. Vayssiere N, Hemm S, Zanca M, et al. Magnetic resonance imaging stereotactic target localization for deep brain stimulation in dystonic children. J Neurosurg 2000;93:784–90.

103. Krack P, Dostrovsky J, Ilinsky I, et al. Surgery of the motor thalamus: problems with the present nomenclatures. Mov Disord 2002;17(Suppl 3):S2–8.

104. Deoni SC, Josseau MJ, Rutt BK, et al. Visualization of thalamic nuclei on high resolution, multi-averaged T1 and T2 maps acquired at 1.5 T. Hum Brain Mapp 2005;25:353–9.

105. Deoni SC, Rutt BK, Parrent AG, et al. Segmentation of thalamic nuclei using a modified k-means clustering algorithm and high-resolution quantitative magnetic resonance imaging at 1.5 T. Neuroimage 2007;34:117–26.

106. Mercado R, Mandat T, Moore GR, et al. Three-tesla magnetic resonance imaging of the ventrolateral thalamus: a correlative anatomical description. J Neurosurg 2006;105:279–83.

107. Spiegelmann R, Nissim O, Daniels D, et al. Stereotactic targeting of the ventrointermediate nucleus of the thalamus by direct visualization with high-field MRI. Stereotact Funct Neurosurg 2006;84:19–23.

108. Plaha P, Ben-Shlomo Y, Patel NK, et al. Stimulation of the caudal zona incerta is superior to stimulation of the subthalamic nucleus in improving contralateral parkinsonism. Brain 2006;129: 1732–47.

109. Plaha P, Filipovic S, Gill SS. Induction of parkinsonian resting tremor by stimulation of the caudal zona incerta nucleus: a clinical study. J Neurol Neurosurg Psychiatry 2008;79:514–21.

110. Plaha P, Khan S, Gill SS. Bilateral stimulation of the caudal zona incerta nucleus for tremor control. J Neurol Neurosurg Psychiatry 2008;79:504–13.

111. Pahapill PA, Lozano AM. The pedunculopontine nucleus and Parkinson's disease. Brain 2000; 123(Pt 9):1767–83.

112. Nieuwenhuys R, Van Huijzen C, Voogd J. The human central nervous system: a synopsis and atlas. Berlin: Springer; 1988.

113. Olszweski J, Baxter D. Cytoarchitecture of the human brain stem. Switzerland: Karger; 1982.

114. Paxinos G, Huang XF. Atlas of the human brainstem. San Diego (CA): Academic Press; 1995.

115. Mazzone P, Lozano A, Stanzione P, et al. Implantation of human pedunculopontine nucleus: a safe and clinically relevant target in Parkinson's disease. Neuroreport 2005;16:1877–81.

116. Plaha P, Gill SS. Bilateral deep brain stimulation of the pedunculopontine nucleus for Parkinson's disease. Neuroreport 2005;16:1883–7.

117. Stefani A, Lozano AM, Peppe A, et al. Bilateral deep brain stimulation of the pedunculopontine and subthalamic nuclei in severe Parkinson's disease. Brain 2007;130:1596–607.

118. Galati S, Scarnati E, Mazzone P, et al. Deep brain stimulation promotes excitation and inhibition in subthalamic nucleus in Parkinson's disease. Neuroreport 2008;19:661–6.

119. Yelnik J. PPN or PPD, what is the target for deep brain stimulation in Parkinson's disease? Brain 2007;130:e79, author reply e80.

120. Zrinzo L, Zrinzo LV, Hariz M. The pedunculopontine and peripeduncular nuclei: a tale of two structures. Brain 2007;130:e73, author reply e74.

121. Zrinzo L, Zrinzo LV, Hariz M. The peripeduncular nucleus: a novel target for deep brain stimulation? Neuroreport 2007;18:1301–2.

122. Zrinzo L, Zrinzo LV, Tisch S, et al. Stereotactic localization of the human pedunculopontine nucleus: atlas-based coordinates and validation of a magnetic resonance imaging protocol for direct localization. Brain 2008;131:1588–98.

123. Astrom M, Zrinzo LU, Tisch S, et al. Method for patient-specific finite element modeling and simulation of deep brain stimulation. Med Biol Eng Comput 2009;47:21–8.

124. Lujan JL, Chaturvedi A, McIntyre CC. Tracking the mechanisms of deep brain stimulation for neuropsychiatric disorders. Front Biosci 2008;13: 5892–904.

125. McIntyre CC, Butson CR, Maks CB, et al. Optimizing deep brain stimulation parameter selection with detailed models of the electrode-tissue interface. Conf Proc IEEE Eng Med Biol Soc 2006;1: 893–5.

126. Sedrak M, Gorgulho A, De Salles AF, et al. The role of modern imaging modalities on deep brain stimulation targeting for mental illness. Acta Neurochir Suppl 2008;101:3–7.

127. Aravamuthan BR, Muthusamy KA, Stein JF, et al. Topography of cortical and subcortical connections of the human pedunculopontine and subthalamic nuclei. Neuroimage 2007;37:694–705.

128. Muthusamy KA, Aravamuthan BR, Kringelbach ML, et al. Connectivity of the human pedunculopontine nucleus region and diffusion tensor imaging in surgical targeting. J Neurosurg 2007;107:814–20.

129. Owen SL, Heath J, Kringelbach ML, et al. Preoperative DTI and probabilistic tractography in an amputee with deep brain stimulation for lower limb stump pain. Br J Neurosurg 2007;21:485–90.

130. Breit S, LeBas JF, Koudsie A, et al. Pretargeting for the implantation of stimulation electrodes into the subthalamic nucleus: a comparative study of magnetic resonance imaging and ventriculography. Neurosurgery 2006;58:ONS83–95.

131. Patel NK, Plaha P, Gill SS. Magnetic resonance imaging-directed method for functional neurosurgery using implantable guide tubes. Neurosurgery 2007;61:358–65.

132. Pinsker MO, Herzog J, Falk D, et al. Accuracy and distortion of deep brain stimulation electrodes on postoperative MRI and CT. Zentralbl Neurochir 2008;69:144–7.

133. West J, Fitzpatrick JM, Wang MY, et al. Comparison and evaluation of retrospective intermodality brain image registration techniques. J Comput Assist Tomogr 1997;21:554–66.

134. Fiegele T, Feuchtner G, Sohm F, et al. Accuracy of stereotactic electrode placement in deep brain stimulation by intraoperative computed tomography. Parkinsonism Relat Disord 2008;14:595–9.

135. Yelnik J, Damier P, Demeret S, et al. Localization of stimulating electrodes in patients with Parkinson disease by using a three-dimensional atlas-magnetic resonance imaging coregistration method. J Neurosurg 2003;99:89–99.

136. Ferroli P, Franzini A, Marras C, et al. A simple method to assess accuracy of deep brain stimulation electrode placement: pre-operative stereotactic CT + postoperative MR image fusion. Stereotact Funct Neurosurg 2004;82:14–9.

137. Hamid NA, Mitchell RD, Mocroft P, et al. Targeting the subthalamic nucleus for deep brain stimulation: technical approach and fusion of pre- and

postoperative MR images to define accuracy of lead placement. J Neurol Neurosurg Psychiatry 2005;76:409–14.

138. Pollo C, Villemure JG, Vingerhoets F, et al. Magnetic resonance artifact induced by the electrode Activa 3389: an in vitro and in vivo study. Acta Neurochir (Wien) 2004;146:161–4.

139. Pollo C, Vingerhoets F, Pralong E, et al. Localization of electrodes in the subthalamic nucleus on magnetic resonance imaging. J Neurosurg 2007;106:36–44.

140. Schrader B, Hamel W, Weinert D, et al. Documentation of electrode localization. Mov Disord 2002; 17(Suppl 3):S167–74.

141. Tisch S, Limousin P, Rothwell JC, et al. Changes in forearm reciprocal inhibition following pallidal stimulation for dystonia. Neurology 2006;66:1091–3.

142. Zrinzo L, van Hulzen ALJ, Gorgulho AA, et al. Avoiding the ventricle: a simple step that improves accuracy of anatomical targeting during deep brain stimulation. J Neurosurg 2009;110(6):1283–90.

143. Kondziolka D. Functional radiosurgery. Neurosurgery 1999;44:12–20.

144. Friehs GM, Park MC, Goldman MA, et al. Stereotactic radiosurgery for functional disorders. Neurosurg Focus 2007;23:E3.

145. Matharu M, May A. Functional and structural neuroimaging in trigeminal autonomic cephalalgias. Curr Pain Headache Rep 2008;12:132–7.

146. May A. The contribution of functional neuroimaging to primary headaches. Neurol Sci 2004; 25(Suppl 3):S85–8.

147. Mayberg HS, Lozano AM, Voon V, et al. Deep brain stimulation for treatment-resistant depression. Neuron 2005;45:651–60.

148. Franzini A, Ferroli P, Leone M, et al. Stimulation of the posterior hypothalamus for treatment of chronic intractable cluster headaches: first reported series. Neurosurgery 2003;52:1095–9.

149. Franzini A, Leone M, Messina G, et al. Neuromodulation in treatment of refractory headaches. Neurol Sci 2008;29(Suppl 1):S65–8.

150. Arantes PR, Cardoso EF, Barreiros MA, et al. Performing functional magnetic resonance imaging in patients with Parkinson's disease treated with deep brain stimulation. Mov Disord 2006;21:1154–62.

151. Grafton ST, Turner RS, Desmurget M, et al. Normalizing motor-related brain activity: subthalamic nucleus stimulation in Parkinson disease. Neurology 2006;66:1192–9.

152. Karimi M, Golchin N, Tabbal SD, et al. Subthalamic nucleus stimulation-induced regional blood flow responses correlate with improvement of motor signs in Parkinson disease. Brain 2008; 131(Pt 10):2710–9.

153. Strafella AP, Lozano AM, Ballanger B, et al. rCBF changes associated with PPN stimulation in a patient with Parkinson's disease: a PET study. Mov Disord 2008;23:1051–4.

154. Henderson JM, Tkach J, Phillips M, et al. Permanent neurological deficit related to magnetic resonance imaging in a patient with implanted deep brain stimulation electrodes for Parkinson's disease: case report. Neurosurgery 2005;57: E1063 [discussion: E1063].

155. Spiegel J, Fuss G, Backens M, et al. Transient dystonia following magnetic resonance imaging in a patient with deep brain stimulation electrodes for the treatment of Parkinson disease. Case report. J Neurosurg 2003;99:772–4.

156. Tremmel J, editor. Urgent device correction - change of safe limits for MRI procedures used with medtronic activa deep brain stimulation systems. Minneapolis (MN): Medtronic Inc; 2005.

157. Larson PS, Richardson RM, Starr PA, et al. Magnetic resonance imaging of implanted deep brain stimulators: experience in a large series. Stereotact Funct Neurosurg 2008;86:92–100.

158. Rezai AR, Finelli D, Nyenhuis JA, et al. Neurostimulation systems for deep brain stimulation: in vitro evaluation of magnetic resonance imaging-related heating at 1.5 Tesla. J Magn Reson Imaging 2002;15:241–50.

159. Finelli DA, Rezai AR, Ruggieri PM, et al. MR imaging-related heating of deep brain stimulation electrodes: in vitro study. AJNR Am J Neuroradiol 2002;23:1795–802.

160. Carmichael DW, Pinto S, Limousin-Dowsey P, et al. Functional MRI with active, fully implanted, deep brain stimulation systems: safety and experimental confounds. Neuroimage 2007;37: 508–17.

Index

Note: Page numbers of article titles are in **boldface** type.

A

Ataxia, parkinsonism, orofacial dyskinesia, and dysautonomia, case of, neuroimaging in, 116–118

B

Basal ganglia, echogenicity of, 91–92
Bilateral action tremor, jaw-opening dystonia, and dysarthria, case of, neuroimaging in, 118–120
BOLD-fMRI analysis, for understanding of brain, 108
BOLD hemodynamic response function, predicted, 103, 104
Brain, functional imaging of, PET and functional MRI for, 133–134
　magnetic resonance imaging of, techniques in diagnosis of Parkinsonian syndromes, **29–55**
　techniques of, 30–31
　MR features in, in neurodegenerative parkinsonism, 48, 49
　MR imaging of, safety issues in, 134
　structures of, echogenicity of, causes of, 92
　understanding of, BOLD-fMRI analysis for, 108
Brain stimulation, deep, and MR imaging, 127
　implanted system, 127, 128
　neuroimaging of, 83–84
Brainstem, mesencephalic, sonographic features of, 89–91

C

Cerebellar tremors, 83
Cerebral demyelination, multifocal and diffuse, causes of, 73
Cerebral vascular lesions, detection of, imaging protocol for, 71
Cognitive decline, dysarthria, dystonia, and spastic gait, case of, neuroimaging in, 112–113
　orolingual dyskinia, palatal tremor, and dystonia of legs, case of, neuroimaging in, 113–114
Cognitive impairment, and cerebellar ataxia, case of, neuroimaging in, 115–116
Corticobasal degeneration, pathology of, 60–61

D

DaTSCAN, in essential tremor, 77, 78
　in Holmes tremor syndrome, 80, 81
Dementia with Lewy bodies, clinical features of, 63–64
　diagnosis of, 64

Depression, transcranial B-mode sonography in, 95
Diffusion tensor imaging, of subthalamic nucleus, 21–22
Diffusion-weighted and diffusion tensor imaging, in atypical parkinsonism, studies of, 35, 36–47
　in diagnosis of neurodegenerative Parkinsonian syndromes, 34–35
Diffusion-weighted imaging, in substantia nigra, 13–15
Drug addiction, parkinsonism, early gait instability, and falls in, case of, neuroimaging in, 114–115
Drug-induced tremors, 79
Dystonia, functional imaging in, 107
　possible cause of, 106
　primary, 106
　structural imaging of brain in, 107
　transcranial B-mode sonography in, in dystonia, 97
Dystonic tremor syndromes, 79

E

Electrode placement, in functional neurosurgery, 132–133
Encephalopathy, ephedronic, 115
　manganic, 115
Essential tremor. See *Tremor, essential.*
Extrapyramidal syndromes, PET and SPECT in, **57–68**

F

Functional MRI, clinical indications of, to diagnose neurologic movement disorders, 105
　data analysis, 104–105
　experimental designs in, 104, 105
　findings in select movement disorders, 105–108
　future directions for, 108–109
　in diagnosis of movement disorders, **103–110**
　in essential tremor, 107
　in studies of Parkinson disease, 106
　techniques of, overview of, 103–104
Functional neuroimaging. See *Neuroimaging, functional.*
Functional neurosurgery. See *Neurosurgery, functional.*

G

Gait difficulty, frequent falls, akinetic rigidity, and hypophonic speech, case of, neuroimaging in, 118, 119

doi:10.1016/S1052-5149(09)00124-5

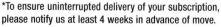

Printed and bound by CPI Group (UK) Ltd, Croydon, CR0 4YY

03/10/2024

01040362-0013